Nona

D1669095

HUNDREDS OF INCREDIBLE RECIPES, SCORES OF TEMPTING MENUS

The renowned Dr. Atkins has now added variety to his revolutionary *diet* . . . by introducing delectable gourmet recipes you never dreamed you would find in a reducing plan!

Would you believe you can now lose weight while eating such delicacies as: Manicotti, Macaroni, Cheese, Coconut Cream Pie, Peanut Butter Cookies or Chocolate Fudge?

Here are hundreds of sumptuous recipes that will make your taste buds come alive, such as Blue Cheese Steak, Cannelloni with Chicken, Broiled Lobster Tails with Tarragon, Skewered Shrimp and Bacon, Creamy Mushroom Soup, Crab-Stuffed Avocado, Chocolate Rum Charlotte, Coffee Cream Layer Cake, Strawberry Ice Cream and many, many, many more!

The cook book millions of low-carbohydrate dieters are waiting for . . .

DR. ATKINS' DIET COOK BOOK

Bantam Books in the Dr. Atkins Diet Series

DR. ATKINS' DIET REVOLUTION by Robert C. Atkins, M.D.

DR. ATKINS' DIET COOK BOOK by Fran Gare and Helen Monica

Dr. Atkins' Diet Cook Book

by FRAN GARE and HELEN MONICA

under the supervision and with an introduction by
ROBERT C. ATKINS, M.D.

BANTAM BOOKS · TORONTO · NEW YORK · LONDON

*This low-priced Bantam Book
has been completely reset in a type face
designed for easy reading, and was printed
from new plates. It contains the complete
text of the original hard-cover edition.*
NOT ONE WORD HAS BEEN OMITTED.

DR. ATKINS' DIET COOK BOOK

*A Bantam Book / published by arrangement with
Crown Publishers, Inc.*

PRINTING HISTORY

Crown edition published June 1974

An excerpt appeared in LADIES' HOME JOURNAL *June 1974*

Bantam edition / May 1975

2nd printing .... June 1975	7th printing .... June 1977
3rd printing .... July 1975	8th printing .... July 1977
4th printing .... February 1976	9th printing .... October 1977
5th printing .... April 1976	10th printing .. December 1977
6th printing .... August 1976	11th printing .... June 1978
12th printing .... June 1979	

*Bantam Books are published by Bantam Books, Inc. Its trade-
mark, consisting of the words "Bantam Books" and the por-
trayal of a bantam, is Registered in U.S. Patent and Trademark
Office and in other countries. Marca Registrada. Bantam
Books, Inc., 666 Fifth Avenue, New York, New York 10019.*

PRINTED IN THE UNITED STATES OF AMERICA

CONTENTS

It is with great warmth and affection that we thank our friend and inspiration Dr. Robert Atkins for allowing us to work with him.

To Shelley Abend, Frank Cohen, Mort Farber, Ernest Ash, Ted Wolcoff, Len Turken, Judy Klopp, Margie O'Donnell, Henrietta Rhein, Donna Putney, Gertha Bernier, Annie Gaskin, thank you for your time and cooperation.

For their love, we thank Corbett Monica and Ivan Gare.

For their patience, our children Tony, Anita, Julie, Nannette, Corby, Elena Monica, and David and Marc Gare.

ROBERT C. ATKINS, M.D.

In our culture the overweight are unattractive. Because they are unhealthy too, most doctors urge the obese to lose weight; yet, rather than health, it is the cosmetic effect that causes them to heed the urging. Both our knowledge of medical statistics and our own personal observations tell the same sad tale—if and when corpulent individuals do lose weight, they very rarely manage to keep it off. Glib-talking medicos refer to most of the overweight as Yo-Yos, but we can't all be Yo-Yos; perhaps we are being criticized rather than given a workable answer to our problem.

We have been brainwashed into believing that *there is only one way* to lose unwanted pounds—by reducing the caloric content of our meals, a painful, hunger-provoking ordeal demanding that we spend the rest of our lives eating *less* than enough to make us physically comfortable. That caloric restriction can control obesity in many people is, of course, so, but that it is the *only* way is blatantly untrue.

Certainly, by now, millions have learned from their own personal experiences that there is an alternative to starvation and semistarvation programs; they have learned that by eliminating most of the carbohydrates

1

that their bodies have been unable to handle (metabolize) properly they not only lost excess weight, but eliminated the curse of hunger, and experienced an upsurge of energy and an exhilarating sense of physical and emotional well-being, a phenomenon rarely observed among low-calorie dieters.

The program they have followed was first described in full detail in *Dr. Atkins' Diet Revolution*. The book became a nationwide best seller for one reason: The diet worked. And it worked better, and longer, and with happier results than any other diet proposal that had heretofore been offered to the public.

Successful dieters compared notes, told one another of their successes, and the fame of the Diet Revolution spread through the grass roots by word of mouth. One told another of losing weight while eating rich, satisfying meals derived from the sumptuous meal plans and recipes that the book provided. But, if *Diet Revolution* was such a success, and its recipes were so acceptable, why is there a need for a menu-cookbook such as this? The answer to that lies in the dieter's need for a practical follow-up program that goes beyond a limited number of recipes, a program recognizing that maintenance of weight loss can only be achieved if the dieter finds enough interest and variety on his diet menu to *want* to live with it indefinitely.

The fact is that far too many people still think of a diet as merely a way to lose weight, a project to be abandoned when the pound-loss goal is reached. But that is not what a diet is. The word "diet" comes from the Latin *diaeta* and Greek *diaita*, meaning "way of life" or "regimen"; and its first dictionary definition is "what a person or animal usually eats and drinks; daily fare." The people who regard a diet as simply a weight-loss program inevitably learn, after repeated painful experiences, that calling an end to a diet often brings back not only the lost weight but the pre-diet discomforts that accompany all forms of obesity. This is particularly true with respect to the most prevalent form of obesity—that associated with intolerance to carbohydrates. When the carbohydrates-intolerant individual gets off his low-carbohydrate diet he quickly regains the fatigue, depression, and other symptoms characteristic of carbohydrate intolerance right along with his old, unwanted poundage. The point I want to drive home is that when I talk about "diet" I'm not talking about quick weight loss or a couple of weeks on a crash diet. I am talking about a way of life, a regimen, our daily fare.

Weight reduction doesn't mean a thing without its sequel: weight control. And weight control, as distinct from the weight reduction obtained through a crash diet, must be a lifelong objective—not an end in itself or a cosmetic device, but important primarily to the extent that it contributes to good health. As such it can be no on-again-off-again game; it is or should be a health habit. In my experience it is best achieved not by concentrating on calories—but by remembering all the nutritive elements, vitamins, and minerals required for good health. In fact, I believe that any diet should be augmented by supplementary vitamins and minerals, not because of the inadequacy of the particular diet, but rather because of the values to be derived from these essential nutrients. Fundamentally I am recommending this type of eating so that you can enjoy good health and a feeling of well-being, keep your weight down while at the same time avoiding hunger.

Avoiding hunger is a very important part of this diet. Obviously to have lasting appeal, the diet must be diverse, and there must be plenty to choose from. An introductory set of recipes will not satisfy many. A way-of-life diet must, to be satisfying as well as effective, be not only nutritious but substantial, flexible, interesting, and, indeed, luxurious. Therefore, this book. If a cookbook can have a theme, this one does. The theme is that dieting is not to be thought of as a brief adventure but as a lifelong practice; not as a painful experience but as a constant pleasure.

It occurs to me that many of you may be wondering

about my statement that the most prevalent form of obesity is that associated with intolerance to carbohydrates. Perhaps you're thinking something of this sort: "Now that's not what I've been taught. Surely most obesity doesn't come from carbohydrate intolerance; it comes from overeating—*calories*. Those of us who overeat will get fat, and those of us who don't will stay slim. All we have to do to lose weight is to learn to eat fewer calories than we burn up. So why shouldn't our diet contain carbohydrates, if we like them, so long as we cut down on the calories?"

That was the thinking before the Diet Revolution, and still is the thinking of those who remain skeptical of its pragmatic applications. It is perfectly true that if you overindulge in all kinds of foods containing all kinds of calories you are going to—unless your metabolism is of the "can't gain" variety—get fat. It is also quite true that reducing the number of calories below the number expended by the body will result in a weight loss. Unfortunately, many people find that they cannot lose weight—or at best can lose it only temporarily—by agonizing calorie-cutting. Massive calorie-cutting is a drastic and self-defeating measure. It isn't usually possible voluntarily to maintain a severely restrictive diet over an extended period of time. Neither is it healthy. Starvation diets are often accompanied by unpleasant side effects and frequently have unpleasant consequences. No, it can no longer be accepted that the way to lose weight is to cut down on the overall intake of calories. Calories count, yes, but some calories count more than others. And obesity *does* result from overeating—but in largest part, from *overeating carbohydrate calories*.

The concept that most obesity results from our inability to deal with the carbohydrates in our diet has the backing of some indisputable scientific findings. We find elevated insulin levels in nearly all obese subjects, elevated triglyceride levels in nearly half, diabetes in the majority, and low blood sugar in the majority. When these carbohydrate-intolerant subjects are placed on a calorie-restricted diet that does allow significant amounts of carbohydrates, they do not do as well as on a carbohydrate-restricted diet. For control of body weight, without the adverse consequences to health and the sense of malaise induced by sharp calorie-cutting and starvation, the reduction of carbohydrates in the diet is by far the more practical, the more acceptable, the more effective, and the more agreeable, lasting way.

All of which brings me back to a sad truth that has always been known but seldom if ever coped with by diet planners: Diets that rely on overall calorie-cutting not only leave you hungry but can be very boring. Perhaps you've had this experience with previous diets, and you recognize that your natural desire for variety can result in your gaining back lost pounds. But there's no need for you to get bored on a well-planned low-carbohydrate diet. Keeping in mind the literally universal need for both substance and variety, we decided to provide additional low-carbohydrate recipes of the kind my patients and readers reported they enjoyed, recipes that will not only help you continue to lose weight if you need to but will also maintain your weight loss. Because if you've already trimmed your body down, you'll want to keep it in good shape while staying in good health.

Fran Gare and Helen Monica, the two homemakers who collaborated on the recipes for the original book and on the present effort, spent years developing these unique menus. Theirs was a challenging task, because of the extremely low level of carbohydrate allotted to each recipe in order to guarantee that no recipe interfere with the effectiveness of the diet, but their success proves that diet food doesn't have to be dull food. I believe that this book will prove to be an invaluable aid to the lifelong dieter or any other truly weight-conscious person, because it provides the know-how for anyone wishing to lead the low-carbohydrate life and enjoy the varied and luxurious cuisine that a low-carbohydrate diet inherently offers. There is enough depth and variety in the following meal plans so that a lifetime of dieting can be achieved without the monotony and boredom that sabotage so many diets. If you are interested in keeping your weight down, and feeling well and eating well throughout your life, this is the cookbook for you.

Since this is not in itself a diet book but a cookbook stressing weight maintenance and designed to provide my reader-dieters with something to get their teeth into even after the thrill of initial weight loss has lost its charm, I do not intend in these pages to spell out all the principles and precepts of the total diet program as enlarged upon in *Dr. Atkins' Diet Revolution*. Reading that book will help you understand this one more thoroughly. But for the benefit of new readers, whether dieters or cookbook collectors, I feel I must explain the basics of The Diet and how it should be used, why it is more than a weight-loss diet, and what I mean by "diet revolution."

In brief: On this diet you don't *watch calories*, you *watch carbohydrates;* you don't *count calories*, and you don't even have to count carbohydrates unless you like counting—you just *don't have any* until a simple test tells you that you are ready for a few, and then you keep them at a level that is specific to *you*. Thus, you don't get stuck in the rut of a rigid dieting regime; you vary it according to your progress. Further: you eat as much as it takes to avoid hunger; you don't get hungry—or, if you do, you eat more; and you never go off your "diet." You adjust it to a maintenance level after you've achieved your weight loss, yes, but you never go off it.

Skeptics have claimed that the diet works by suppressing the appetite and thus decreasing the intake of calories. This is only partially true, because most people find they *do* eat fewer calories when carbohydrates are sharply restricted. But it does provide a "metabolic advantage," which allows many dieters to eat and enjoy thousands of calories, of the noncarbohydrate variety of course. At the same time one of its great advantages is that, while it does not "suppress" the appetite, it does indeed control the pathologic hunger and abnormally excessive appetite that is such a common clinical finding in overweight individuals. So dramatic is this benefit that the most distressing of all clinical appetite disorders—namely, the night-eating syndrome—can be halted with just three words: "Stop eating carbohydrates."

Through painstaking personal supervision of ten thousand obese patients, I have found that cutting carbohydrates down to a level that approaches "biologic zero" will place one on the most efficient diet I have ever observed. "Biologic zero," you will need to know, translates into "zero for all practical purposes." In other words, it "will provide the same response as if it were zero." Quite a number of foods that we don't ordinarily think of as sources of carbohydrates actually contain 1 or 2 grams of carbohydrates; so that even on the strictest "zero" level, we have found we are consuming around 10 grams per day. On this diet you will not only lose weight by logically correcting for your carbohydrate intolerance, · but you will feel an improvement in well-being and an upsurge of energy due in large part to the reduction of carbohydrates and the natural biologic adjustments your body makes. After one brief encounter with dieting at this low-low-carbohydrate level, I'm sure you'll be convinced of its value—that you'll be ready and eager to join the Diet Revolution and keep those carbohydrates *down*. Not permanently down to zero, as you will discover, but way down.

One key to understanding the value of a near zero carbohydrate diet is to understand the role of ketone bodies in human metabolism. You may have heard some critics exclaim that ketosis (the word used to describe the condition of the metabolism when these basic body chemicals are found in the body) is dangerous and must be avoided. Well, these ketone bodies are anything but dangerous; they are vital metabolic fuel that serve a critically important function for the body. At least 95 percent of the fuel we carry in our bodies is in the form of stored fat, which is usually released into the bloodstream as free fatty acids, which are powerful energy sources to the body's tissues, yet cannot reach the brain for its vital functions. But the brain can and does use these ketone bodies in greater amounts even than it uses glucose, the fuel it uses when carbohydrates are present in the diet.

So when you are "in ketosis," all it means is that your body is functioning quite nicely, using a valuable fuel of metabolism that comes from the very source you hope to use up—if you are trying to slim down— the fat you have stored in your body. This only occurs during those times of your life when your body's carbo- hydrate (glycogen) stores are low and thus the bio- logically zero diet becomes referred to as the ketogenic diet.

Another key to understanding the effects of carbo- hydrate restriction lies in understanding the role that insulin plays in the body. Insulin is a very valuable hormone because it serves the important function of processing the glucose in the blood into energy that we can use for the functions of life. But when it exists in excess, as it does in virtually every significantly over- weight individual, then it can convert this glucose into fat and, moreover, it can prevent the breakdown of fat in the body so that the individual has difficulty in losing weight. The Diet is therefore geared to diminish the excessive insulin response that is the hall- mark of the overweight. But how does The Diet do it? You may wonder. Well, the intake of carbohydrates stimulates the production of insulin; and in the vast number of obese individuals who demonstrate a degree of carbohydrate intolerance—that is, an abnormality in carbohydrate metabolism—the carbohydrates taken in, whether or not they would be considered excessive under conditions of normal metabolism, stimulate an overproduction of insulin. Think of it in the simplest of all possible terms: Carbohydrates release insulin, which converts glucose into fat. This may not satisfy the medical purists, but you will have gotten the idea.

Traditional theories in which calorie-is-a-calorie-is-a-calorie do not take into account the disturbance in insulin balance exhibited by the overweight individual, even though it is well known that carbohydrates call for the greatest and most immediate insulin release on the part of the dieter. Tradition shouldn't be treated as Holy Writ. There is room for new thinking on the dietary scene.

The action of the ultralow-carbohydrate diet in stabilizing the insulin levels and thereby stabilizing the blood sugar levels can perhaps bring about one of the most valuable side benefits a dieter can hope to experience. Low blood sugar levels—or, more precisely, fluctuating or unstable blood sugar levels—are, in my observation, really common to a majority of people in our modern society. The overwhelming majority of ketogenic dieters report an increased sense of well-being, which in my view is a result of the stabilization of blood sugar levels effected by the low-low-carbohydrate intake. Certainly, the majority of my patients and thousands of readers have told me personally that they actually felt an upsurge of energy and an improvement in mental outlook after making drastic cuts of the carbohydrates in their diets. This phenomenon in which the *removal* of quick energy foods creates an *increase* in physical energy is, in my opinion, caused by the correction of low blood sugar (hypoglycemia). Perhaps this concept can be more readily understood if I say that quick energy is not lasting energy, and that a blood sugar level quickly raised is quickly dropped. Thus, the innumerable people who are affected by the problem of hypoglycemia do experience an increased feeling of well-being when they eliminate carbohydrates, the quick-energy foods that leave fatigue in their wake.

One cannot talk about low blood sugar without progressing to the subject of vitamins.

It has been said that if a diet requires vitamins, that is prima facie evidence that it is nutritionally inadequate. But this is unsophisticated, even simplistic, thinking. Most every physician working with hypoglycemia soon learns through clinical experience that megadosages of vitamins in the B complex family and vitamins C and E are of extreme clinical value in improving the various physical and mental complaints that accompany low blood sugar. In recognizing the high percentage of overweight people who have low blood sugar, it is not difficult to see why megavitamins are of enormous value in the management of overweight patients.

When I first began to work with this diet I used only an ordinary vitamin and mineral supplement, but the years of experience have taught me the value of increased dosages and I'd like to pass my recommendation on to you. No more than standard doses of A and D should be taken, because these are fat-soluble and have the capacity to store up within the body (to toxicity levels) if taken in chronic excess, but the entire spectrum of the B complex as well as C and E vitamins should be taken in significant dosages along with minerals such as calcium and magnesium.*

As I review the years of my practice, I can clearly see the great benefits of the stepped-up use of these vitamins and minerals. I have come to believe that they are an integral part not only of the Diet Revolution program but probably of any diet. I think it is likely that if one examined the eating patterns in most parts of our country, one would see that many of these nutrients are in short supply in our daily fare regardless of whether or not we are dieting. Therefore it is

* I recommend a multiple high potency vitamin, an adequate supply of multiple mineral tablets, 1500 milligrams of vitamin C, and 800 units of vitamin E for an average patient, the dosage being regulated upward or downward according to the needs or tolerance of the individual patient based on his physician's recommendations. B complex has proven to be of great value to many individuals who manifest some degree of fatigue, which I like to give in a formula providing 50 milligrams of all subconstituents two or three times a day.

not surprising to find that the addition of these dietary elements often provides a measurable improvement in the state of well-being. Thus, when people ask me to explain why my patients show an improvement in physical condition and mental outlook on this diet when previous studies seem to indicate indifferent, equivocal, or sometimes detrimental results from various types of low-carbohydrate diets, I have to say that one reason is the recommended supplement. It works hand in glove with the principles of carbohydrate restriction and the stabilization of low blood sugar.

With the understanding of two key biologic principles—one, that virtually all obese individuals demonstrate some degree of carbohydrate intolerance, and two, that there is a wide degree of individual variation of biologic responses, you can quickly learn the principles of the Diet Revolution. If you consult the book of that name, in which I present my complete game-plan for sustained weight loss, you will learn a simple method by which you can determine, for yourself, your own Critical Carbohydrate Level, or CCL —that level or quantity of carbohydrate intake below which you have to stay in order to ensure sustained weight loss, continued health and biochemical improvement, and that great sense of feeling good. With this understanding you can tailor your diet to your own metabolic response as well as your food preferences and life-style.

You will note that there is a difference between "critical carbohydrate level" and "zero carbohydrate level." The critical level is somewhere above zero and varies from individual to individual. What we have here is, in effect, a bonus for successful and sustained weight loss. Everyone who has followed the *Diet Revolution* weight-loss plan knows that the initial weight loss is usually very rapid and goes on being rapid—especially if there's a lot of weight to lose—so long as the dieter sticks to, or close to, the ketogenic level. They know, and as you too will realize on browsing through the recipes in this book, that it is quite unnecessary to be bound to zero carbohydrate for life.

In fact, with the occasional exception of a particularly difficult obesity case, it is unnecessary to remain at zero carbohydrate for more than a few days. Now if you think I'm contradicting my basic premise of an ultra-low-carbohydrate diet, take a closer look at the recipes. You'll see that each of them has been allocated two carbohydrate counts: a total gram count for the entire quantity and a gram count per serving, that is, your share of the recipe. In some cases the count per serving is very close to zero, and in others it is not so close. You may note instances of 4, 5, and 6 gram servings. Maybe you'll even have such meals three times a day, approaching a day's total of 15 or 20 grams. This, in terms of zero carbohydrate, is quite high. But when compared to the non-ketogenic low-carbohydrate diets, where 50 or 60 grams are allowed, it is still rather strict.

The purpose of introducing small quantities of carbohydrate into the regimen is something I explain in considerable detail in the original diet book and so will only summarize briefly at this stage: Having found that the loss in weight and the gain in well-being is so great in the initial phase of the diet, I gradually add —for variety, for menu balance, for taste, to prevent excess loss, and particularly to begin to evolve a lifetime maintenance program—small quantities of carbohydrate to the overall daily fare until the individual's cutoff point—the point at which he is on the verge of regaining weight—is reached. This represents the personal Critical Carbohydrate Level. Thus, the basic requirement of this lifelong dietary regimen is for you to keep track of your carbohydrate intake: to keep it under control, and not to let it get ahead of your capacity to handle it.

I am often asked what is "new" and "revolutionary" about the Diet Revolution weight reduction program and how it differs from other low-carbohydrate diets. Well, of course, the idea of "cutting down" on carbohydrates is *not* new. But the book does call for a revolution in our thinking, a recognition that calories of different origins have different effects in the body and that the traditional "balanced" diet has one drawback for the obese individual—it contains too many carbohydrates, and these carbohydrates can make the fat person fatter. Furthermore, this is not just another low-carbohydrate or zero-carbohydrate crash diet. It is a graduated, very-low-carbohydrate diet taken in conjunction with significant dosages of vitamins and minerals, and designed, not simply for weight loss but for optimum weight maintenance and lifelong use.

Critics have pointed out that all the low-carbohydrate diets of the past have faded into obscurity. Why, the doubters ask, have *they* faded if *this* diet works? Again I must say that they were *not* "this diet." The previous diets cannot be accepted as anything more than pioneering steps in the right direction. The Diet Revolution program represents the culmination of a medically sound low-carbohydrate way of life— and once again I repeat, *way of life*—not simply a crash reduction diet. That has always been one of the problems with some of the so-called predecessor diets: Their ephemeral quality, their emphasis on weight loss today and never mind tomorrow. Linked to this is the matter of their definition of "low carbohydrate." It has either been zero, on a crash diet basis, or not nearly low enough to be universally effective. Another problem with the previous diets has been their general disregard of the need for effective vitamin-mineral supplementation, which to me is of prime importance. And yet another problem, in my estimation, has been the lack of variety or interest offered in their diet menus. It is in this connection that I feel the recipes in this book go a long way toward providing the varied and appealing fare that makes a low-low-carbohydrate plan enjoyable and which this diet's sound physiological principles merit.

Thus, The Diet differs from related diets in many ways but among the big differences are these: One, it is not a low-carbohydrate diet, it is a *drastically reduced carbohydrate diet;* two, it is not limited to a period of a few days or a few weeks, it is a lifelong program. It is "daily fare." And it is not daily fare consisting of such old-fashioned diet staples as carrot sticks, watery bouillon, skim milk, celery stalks, or butterless toast. (Toastless butter, yes!) It is daily fare consisting of such stick-to-the-ribs menu items as stuffed steak, creamy mushroom soup, tossed salad with tomato dressing, broiled lobster tails with tarragon, skewered shrimp and bacon, cheese soufflé, beef Stroganoff, moussaka, crab-stuffed avocado, cannelloni with chicken, coconut cream pie, chocolate rum charlotte, and many, many more—made according to the mouth-watering recipes devised by Fran and Helen and described in the pages to follow.

"Aha!" you may think. "You're giving me recipes that *sound* mouth-watering but surely contain substitute ingredients that make them much less delicious than they look."

But no; we're not. Some of the recipes do contain the occasional substitute ingredient, particularly when an artificial sweetener is required; but the purpose of such recipes is to provide you with something that does taste delicious, that will taste like the carbohydrate food you have given up, that will help you fight off any lingering craving you may think you have for a sugary dessert or starchy side dish . . . and do it without the sugar and the starch.

However, most of the recipes in this book do not rely on substitute ingredients of any sort. They rely on ingredients, on natural and nutritious foods, that contain a minimum of carbohydrate. The whole point of the meal plans, the daily fare, offered in the following pages is to provide you with a gourmet's choice of thoroughly palatable meals to live with not just for a few days or a few weeks but for a long, long time— your lifetime. Would you want to live without butter and eggs forever? Without berries and whipped cream? Without mayonnaise? Without creamy soups, salad dressings, pâté? Without fried foods, bacon, blue cheese, Hollandaise sauce? Well, if you're like the majority of my patients, you don't have to. You can live *with* all these things. This diet isn't one that you're going to be tempted to abandon. You will like it; you will want to stay on it for the rest of your life. If you need to lose weight on this diet, you will; if you have already lost your extra pounds and reached your optimal weight, you'll be able to maintain it with ease. (If you don't know your optimal weight—that is, your best weight, in accordance with your height, build, sex, and age—you might refer to one of the many weight charts readily available.) What I want to stress throughout this book is the concept of a nutritional regime for lifelong use—for health, weight maintenance, eating pleasure, and zestful living.

As a physician I must point out that the Diet Revolution is meant to be followed under a doctor's care or management, and it is designed to supplement rather than replace good medical care. I have always insisted on this, but I would like to make doubly clear in these pages that *all* diets should be followed under a doctor's supervision. Of course, one does not have to consult a physician before preparing a few recipes from a cookbook. But he certainly would have to consult one if he were about to change his lifetime eating pattern, which is what I'm recommending for those of you who find weight control a problem. As I have noted, its precepts were tested by careful, meticulous clinical observations on more than ten thousand patients who returned for repeated examination while following The Diet. I have found it incomparably effective; I have found it to be remarkably free of ill effect. The Diet came about through personal trial and error, through experimentation upon myself, through cautious application of tested principles to thousands of very different people, and through careful adaptation to their individual needs. It is the honest distillation of the findings and refinements evolved through years of experience in the medical management of the many overweight individuals who have consulted me.

Nevertheless, the fact is that not all overweight subjects respond to a given diet in the same way. They have their individual differences. A diet that can cause one person to lose weight can cause another to gain. The same diet that can cause one individual's cholesterol level to drop can cause another's to rise. You don't need a doctor to tell you whether or not you're losing weight or whether or not you're feeling well. You're the best judge of that. You don't need a doctor to determine your own height, frame, and musculature, and, from these factors, your own desirable weight. You don't need a doctor to determine whether your diet is suitable for achieving your weight reduction and maintenance objectives, because you can easily employ the self-testing method described in *Diet Revolution*. But you do need a doctor to tell you how you are progressing with your cholesterol, triglyceride, glucose, or uric acid levels, the variables most likely to be affected by The Diet, and which, of course, bear directly upon your health. Of one thing I can assure you: Whenever a disquieting complication has arisen in my experience, it has always been possible to modify The Diet or prescribe appropriate medication. This, of course, cannot be done without the aid of a physician.

There have, in fact, been instances where The Diet has had to be modified, but there are very few general categories where it is absolutely contraindicated. When another medical illness coexists along with obesity, a diet must always be handled in the light of medical expertise and medical judgment. Certainly a person with a medical condition in addition to obesity should not follow The Diet without consulting his physician —one such person, for example, being the insulin-dependent diabetic (and remember, an overwhelming majority of diabetics do not require insulin), and another being a patient with a degree of renal (kidney) failure or insufficiency that demands the restriction of protein. But I have never seen fit to abandon the basic principle of The Diet in managing the case of a person who was overweight, regardless of his complications. For instance, I have managed all my pregnant patients, in cooperation with their obstetricians, with a modified version of this diet, and have had excellent results—both on the part of the mother and the offspring—bearing in mind that the objective during pregnancy is not the loss of weight but the prevention of an undue weight gain. In accomplishing this objective it is not necessary to restrict the carbohydrate level to the bare minimum required by the weight-loss phase of the diet program.

The question of cholesterol in the diet and in the blood has been one of the main issues under medical discussion in regard to this diet. Some physicians are reluctant to recommend a diet that contains unlimited amounts of cholesterol and saturated fats. Their position is that, in individuals who respond with an increase of plasma lipids (fats), the risk of coronary artery disease may be increased. As a physician with significant training in cardiology, I have more than some familiarity with the ailments of the heart. There is no question that a person whose cholesterol level is too high may indeed run an increased risk of heart disease. But it has not been demonstrated that significant elevations of cholesterol or other lipid levels occur with any distressing frequency in overweight individuals following this dietary regimen. My own findings have, in fact, been to the contrary.

There are many factors governing people's blood fat levels, as well as their likelihood for developing heart disease. The amount of saturated fat in the diet is certainly one of the factors; but so, too, is the intake of sugar and other refined carbohydrates. We know of many cultures that have a high fat diet but low cholesterol readings and a low incidence of heart disease. And, conversely, we know of some individuals whose cholesterol levels will go up on a high fat diet, particularly if they cheat by also taking in carbohydrates.

My own records on the effects of The Diet upon the cholesterol and triglyceride levels of my patients indicate that there is an improvement, a lowering of the levels, more often than not. But then, my patients seldom cheat. They find The Diet too satisfying.

Yet each dieter has a personal obligation to make sure that he is not in the group whose cholesterol goes up significantly. This means—and here there can be no compromise—that he must go to a doctor and get blood tests before embarking on The Diet, and again after having been on it for a month or so. Only in this manner can the dieter be sure that he is not one who must restrict, or at least control, the intake of animal fats.

But I do want to point out that an initially high cholesterol does not necessarily mean that a low fat diet must be followed. This is only true in the case of a cholesterol level that rises from its original level while The Diet is being used—a clear indication that The Diet is not properly tailored for the individual and should be modified. For the most part—in fact, with a significant percentage of overweight people initially exhibiting high cholesterol—the cholesterol level will go down by cutting out the carbohydrates without necessarily prohibiting the use of fat.

One of the favorite ploys by critics of The Diet has been to proclaim that it is a high fat diet. Perhaps you will be surprised to learn that it is not. It has been shown that when the intake of carbohydrates is lowered to a rather generous level of 60 grams without calling for any restriction of fat, careful dietary histories show a decrease in the intake of fat by some 20 percent. This is attributed to the elimination from the diet of such items as ice cream, pies, French fries, bread and butter, and so on, and to reduction of appetite and food intake. But on the ketogenic diet we recommend, the loss of appetite is even greater and the intake of fat even lower.

That is one reason we have found that the average patient can include such ingredients as cream, butter, eggs, and cheese, high fat foods that make a recipe so appealing.

But there will still be some individuals who will not respond well to this level of fat intake. If you find that you are such a person, you can easily modify the ketogenic diet so that it is also restricted in fat.

Under the heading "Low Fat Recipes" you will find an assortment of dishes that do precisely this. As you will see, the recipes follow all the principles of this diet, yet include very little fat. At the same time the recipes are attractive enough to interest even those who have no concern about a low fat diet.

In any event, *do* check out your diet plans with your doctor.

But, you may ask, what do I do if my physician is not sympathetic to the theories expounded in the Diet Revolution? Well, I think you will find that the situation is not so discouraging as it was in the past. Most doctors are interested in seeing their patients' health improved and are willing to work with a patient who genuinely wants to do something constructive about it. Explain that you would like him to give you a thorough checkup; that you would want to take blood tests both at this initial stage and at later stages of your diet; and that you will certainly want him to give you periodic examinations to check out, among other things, your uric acid and cholesterol levels.

I believe your doctor, under these circumstances, will be happy to have you try your new diet plan. He will appreciate your determination to take action toward benefiting your health. Your own interest and dedication, coupled with his as your personal physician, will lead to his paying extra careful attention to your progress as you follow The Diet—to your weight loss, your health gain, your new energy, and, in all likelihood, your improvement in blood test values. If he finds that this or any other diet is contraindicated in your case by any medical condition, he will tell you and advise you accordingly. In my experience, as I've said, contraindications for this diet are extremely few, and side effects (occasional accompaniments of any diet, especially if the diet is misapplied) are rare and are usually cleared up without difficulty.

Still, I must stress that any basic change in eating habits should not be made without medical advice and periodic checkups. You may be the best judge of how you feel and even of how you look, but your doctor is the best judge of the changes that take place inside. So do ask your personal physician if he is willing to supervise your zero-to-low-carbohydrate plan. You will be surprised at the growing number of doctors who, having observed the benefits of the diet, are beginning to prescribe carbohydrate restriction to their patients.

But this is not really a book about dieting, nor is it a medical treatise. This is a book about food, good food, beautiful food, food that I myself eat to maintain my own weight loss and exuberant good health. It is a cookbook, and a very special one, designed to serve as a supplement to *Dr. Atkins' Diet Revolution*. And the purpose of this cookbook, with its more than 300 new low-low-carbohydrate recipes, is not just to help you lose excess pounds if you still need to lose any; it is primarily to help you maintain the loss once you have achieved your optimum weight.

If you have been following The Diet you will know that it consists of several phases. In the early phases you lose weight rapidly. Quite soon you begin to approach your optimum weight. As you do so you gradually make changes in your menu—small changes, but interesting and satisfying ones. At a certain stage, specific to you as an individual, you reach your best weight. And at this point, something gratifying happens. Your weight stabilizes. Not perfectly, perhaps, but within a range of a few pounds. Now it will not do so if your carbohydrate intake is too low, in which case you will continue to lose some weight; and it will not do so if your carbohydrate intake has crept too high, in which case you will probably regain. But there is an ideal weight for your body structure, and when you reach it on this diet and if you continue to follow the diet plan carefully, you won't make mistakes with your carbohydrate intake and you will not experience a continued weight loss nor an alarming weight gain.

What is the secret of this stabilization of weight? It is your CCL, your Critical Carbohydrate Level. If you keep track of this, as you must, you will never lose too much and you will never gain too much. Preferably, you will not permit your weight to fluctuate at all after you have reached your weight-loss goal, but there is no need for you to worry if it varies one way or the other within five pounds or so. You can always adjust your carbohydrate intake to maintain the balance: Either cut down on the treats or give yourself some extras.

You will see why I continue to refer you to the original diet book. It is a handbook for your complete understanding of the 21-day recipe program that follows in this book. This is not to say that you cannot safely use every single recipe in this book as isolated examples of good low-carbohydrate cookery, but I have always liked my patients and my readers to have full knowledge of what they're being advised to do and why. That's what the *Diet Revolution* handbook is for.

This book is for your continued eating pleasure.

I am sometimes asked: "What is the difference between weight loss and weight maintenance?" "How can a diet that produces weight loss also assure maintenance of that loss?"

Well, it's really quite simple. The diet is flexible. And the recipes in this book demonstrate that flexibility. In the biologic zero phase of the diet plan you lose with some rapidity. As you gradually add small quantities of carbohydrate, you lose more slowly. As you add even more—always keeping track of your CCL—you stabilize; you maintain your weight at an even keel. Watch your scale, watch the gram counts in the recipes, watch your CCL and live by it, and you have the whole simple secret of maintenance.

To appreciate the value of these recipes as part of a maintenance program, you have to realize just how long you are going to be on a diet. By the mere fact of being overweight you have shown that you have a weight problem. This means that, given the freedom to eat according to your body's natural desires, you have every right to expect that your weight will eventually reach its highest point instead of stabilizing at some not-so-overweight level.

In order not to spend your life at your weight's high point, or "high-water mark," you are going to have to accept the fact that proper weight is a matter of lifetime eating habits. Loss of weight might represent only 1 percent of the diet battle. This book is for the maintenance battle—the other 99 percent of your life.

But let me assure you that the maintenance battle, on this diet, is a pleasure. Although I am not myself a gourmet chef and could not have devised the contents of this book in my bachelor kitchen, I can vouch that I have tried many of the recipes and have not found them wanting—or found myself wanting—in any way. I can first of all confirm that the recipes and menus are altogether suitable for the person in normal health who wishes a carefully planned diet with a built-in, appropriately low-carbohydrate level. But I can further state that the recipes make satisfying meals and satisfying taste treats. This is good food. This is luscious food! Spicy spareribs . . . creamy dumplings for soup . . . blue cheese steak . . . deviled-salmon eggs . . . sherry dressing . . . lobster stew . . . gnocchi . . . ham and egg fritters . . . sausage and peppers . . . lemon-lime mousse . . . strawberry parfait. . . !

Let me lead you into a new experience in superb and healthful eating with a hearty—

Bon appétit!

21-DAY RECIPE PROGRAM

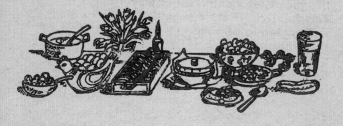

WEEK 1

MONDAY
Breakfast
  *Omelet with a Special
    Taste
  Diet Soda, Coffee, or
    Tea

Lunch
  *Chicken Salad Ham
    Rolls
  1 cup *Dressing of the
    House
  *Orange Cooler

Dinner
  *Spicy Spareribs
  Hearts of Lettuce Salad
    *Blender Dressing
    for Greens
  *Coffee Foam
  Diet Soda, Coffee, or
    Tea

Snack
  *Salmon Salad in a
    Hurry
  Diet Soda

TUESDAY
Breakfast
  *Basic Fluffy Omelet
  Canadian Bacon
  Diet Soda, Coffee, or
    Tea

Lunch
  *Ham and Egg Balls
    with Green Pepper
    Rings and Radishes
  Sour Pickle
  Gelatin
  Diet Soda, Coffee, or
    Tea

Dinner
  Clam Broth
  *Broiled Lobster Tails
    with Tarragon
  Tossed Salad with Oil
    and Vinegar
  *Strawberry Sponge
  Coffee, Tea, or Diet
    Soda

Snack
  *Buttered Radishes
  Green Pepper Rings

WEDNESDAY
Breakfast
  *Cheese Omelet with
    Link Sausages
  Diet Soda, Coffee, or
    Tea

Lunch
  *Skewered Shrimp and
    Bacon
  1 cup salad with *Basic
    French Dressing
  *The "Pop" Pop
  Diet Soda, Coffee, or
    Tea

° These recipes can be found in the text.

Dinner
- *Creamy Dumplings for Soup
- *Lemon Basted Roast Chicken
- Cucumbers marinated in Herbs, Oil, and Vinegar
- *Fruit Mold
- Diet Soda, Coffee, or Tea

Snack
- *Instant Iced Coffee
- *Salami and Parmesan

THURSDAY
Breakfast
- *Shrimp Curry with Eggs
- Diet Soda, Coffee, or Tea

Lunch
- *Stracciatella Soup
- Assorted Cheese Platter
- Prosciutto
- *Coffee Foam
- Espresso

Dinner
- *Blue Cheese Steak
- *Not Just Another Tossed Salad
- *Pink Lady
- Diet Soda, Coffee, or Tea

Snack
- *Swiss Snack
- *Meringue Munchies
- Diet Soda

FRIDAY
Breakfast
- *Peppers and Eggs (substitute 2 eggs for each ½ cup Egg Beaters)
- Diet Soda, Coffee, or Tea

Lunch
- Smoked Whitefish with *Deviled-Salmon Eggs
- Crisp Lettuce Leaves
- *Orange Cooler

Dinner
- *Baked Fish Loaf with *Tartare Sauce
- Tossed Salad
- *Cheese Pudding
- Diet Soda, Coffee, or Tea

Snack
- *Heavenly Wings
- Iced Tea

SATURDAY
Breakfast
- *Rhubarb Snack
- *Orange Cooler
- Diet Soda, Coffee, or Tea

Lunch
- *Quick Bouillon Pickup
- *Bacon and Egg Salad on Endive Leaves
- *Strawberry Sponge
- Diet Soda, Coffee, or Tea

Dinner
- *Luscious Lamb
- Green Pepper Ring and Radishes with *Bacon Cream Sauce
- *Dessert Fritters
- Diet Soda, Coffee, or Tea

Snack
- Salami and Ham Slices
- Assorted Hard Cheeses
- Diet Soda

SUNDAY
Breakfast
- Scrambled Eggs with Ham and *Cheese Sauce
- Diet Soda, Coffee, or Tea

Lunch
- *Cheese It
- *Meringue Munchies
- 1 cup salad with *Sherry Dressing
- *The "Pop" Pop
- Diet Soda, Coffee, or Tea

Dinner
- *Italian Garlic Soup
- *Veal with Tuna Sauce
- Romaine Lettuce with Crisp Bacon and *Dressing of the House
- *Vanilla Ice Cream
- Diet Soda, Coffee, or Tea

Snack
- *Cottage Cheese Dip
- Baken-ets
- Coffee

WEEK 2

MONDAY
Breakfast
- *Fluffy Jam Omelet
- Diet Soda, Coffee, or Tea

Lunch
- *Cottage Cheese Slices on Lettuce Leaves
- *2 Peanut Butter Cookies
- Coffee or Tea

Dinner
- *Cheddar Olives and Celery
- *Gourmet Game Hens
- Vegetable Salad with *Russian Dressing
- *Coconut Cream Pie

Snack
   ¼ cantaloupe
   Iced Tea

TUESDAY
Breakfast
   *Eggs Florentine
   Coffee or Tea

Lunch
   *Cold Spiced Beef
   1 cup Tossed Salad
      with *Our Favorite
      Roquefort Dressing
   *Butterscotch Cream
      Pudding
   Iced Coffee or Tea

Dinner
   *Cheese Balls
   *Broiled Fresh Salmon
   *Cole Slaw Our Way
   *Strawberry Torte
   Diet Soda, Coffee, or
      Tea

Snack
   *Brownies
   *Orange Cooler

WEDNESDAY
Breakfast
   *Cheese Soufflé
   Coffee or Tea

Lunch
   *Seafood and Avocado
      Salad
   *2 Coconut Drops
   Diet Soda, Coffee, or
      Tea

Dinner
   *Creamy Mushroom
      Soup
   *Spiced Black Olives
      tossed with Pimentos
   *Cheddar and Chicken
   *Chocolate Rum
      Charlotte
   Diet Soda, Coffee, or
      Tea

Snack
   *Toasted Almonds
   Diet Soda

THURSDAY
Breakfast
   *Eggs and Swiss Cheese
   *Meringue Munchies
   Coffee or Tea

Lunch
   *Ham Salad Donna
   *Green Bean Salad
   *Blueberry Ice Cream
   Diet Soda, Coffee, or
      Tea

Dinner
   *Italian Garlic Soup
   *Steak Pizzaiola
   *Baked Spinach
   *Coffee Cream Layer
      Cake
   Diet Soda, Coffee, or
      Tea

Snack
   Celery Stuffed with
      *Tuna Delight

FRIDAY
Breakfast
  *Cheese Omelet
  *Meringue Munchies
  Coffee or Tea

Lunch
  *Tuna Surprise
  1 cup salad with
    *Vinaigrette Cream
    Dressing
  *Chocolate Shake

Dinner
  *Lobster Soup
  *Shrimp Scampi
  *The Most Delicious
    Cucumbers
  *Strawberry-Lemon
    Meringue Pie
  *Diet Soda, Coffee, or
    Tea

Snack
  *Instant Iced Coffee
  *Mexican Almonds

SATURDAY
Breakfast
  *Eggs and Asparagus
    with Cream Sauce
  Coffee or Tea

Lunch
  *Roast Beef Salad
  *Cole Slaw Our Way
  *Cottage Cheese
    Custard
  Diet Soda, Coffee, or
    Tea

Dinner
  *Hungarian Veal Stew
  *Radish Relish
  *Gnocchi
  *Strawberry Parfait
  Coffee or Tea

Snack
  Shrimp with *Cocktail
    Sauce
  Diet Soda

SUNDAY
Breakfast
  *Scrambled Eggs in
    Cheese Sauce with
    Sausages
  Coffee or Tea

Lunch
  *Avocado and Spinach
    Salad
  *2 Brownies
  Diet Soda, Coffee, or
    Tea

Dinner
  *Gazpacho
  *Beef Stroganoff
  *String Beans
    Amandine
  *Pretty Ginger Ale
    Mold

Snack
  *Blender-Thick
    Raspberry Shake

WEEK 3

MONDAY
Breakfast
  *Bacon and Onion
    Omelet
  Coffee or Tea

Lunch
  *Cottage Cheese Lime
    Mold
  *Ice Cream Soda

Dinner
  *Onion Soup
  *Salmon à la
    Napolitana
  *Zucchini Stuffed with
    Cream Sauce
  *Chocolate Cream
    Debbie
  Coffee or Tea

Snack
  *Chocolate Almonds
  Diet Soda

TUESDAY
Breakfast
  *Ham and Egg Fritters
  Diet Soda, Coffee, or
    Tea

Lunch
  *Cheese-stuffed
    Eggplant
  *Orange Cooler
  *Coconut Snowflakes
  Coffee or Tea

Dinner
  *Crabmeat Almond Pie
  *Sausage and Peppers
  *Tossed Salad with
    Tomato Dressing
  *Zabaglione
  Diet Soda, Coffee, or
    Tea

Snack
  *Chocolate Shake

WEDNESDAY
Breakfast
  *Mushrooms, Onions,
    and Eggs
  Diet Soda, Coffee, or
    Tea

Lunch
  *Spinach Salad Special
  *Shape-Up Shake

Dinner
  *Stuffed Eggs (Greek
    Style)
  *Greek Salad
  *Moussaka
  *Glazed Strawberries
  Diet Soda, Coffee, or
    Tea

Snack
  *Peanut Butter Dreams
  Diet Soda

THURSDAY
Breakfast
  *Baked Ham Soufflé
  Coffee or Tea

Lunch
- *Crab-stuffed Avocado
- *Cappuccino

Dinner
- *Nutty Cocktail Balls
- *A Pork Chop Meal
- *Mock Potato
  Dumplings
- *Lemon-Lime Mousse
- Diet Soda, Coffee, or
  Tea

Snack
- *Ice Cream Soda
- *Mexican Almonds

FRIDAY
Breakfast
- *Crabmeat and
  Mushroom Omelet
- Coffee or Tea

Lunch
- *Cheese and Onion Pie
- *Zesty Zucchini
- *Strawberry Ice Cream
- Diet Soda, Coffee, or
  Tea

Dinner
- *Senegalese Soup
- *Fabulous Flounder
- *Cauliflower in Cheese
  Sauce
- *Sweet Crepe
- Diet Soda, Coffee, or
  Tea

Snack
- *Hot Chocolate
- Assorted Hard Cheeses
- *Meringue Munchies

SATURDAY
Breakfast
- *Cheese Pancakes
- *Blueberry-Raspberry
  Jelly
- Coffee or Tea

Lunch
- Assorted Cold Cuts
  with Mustard
- *Mock Potato Salad
- *Cantaloupe and Wine
- Diet Soda, Coffee, or
  Tea

Dinner
- *Stuffed Mushrooms
- *Cannelloni with
  Chicken
- *Asparagus with
  Parmesan Cheese
- *Macadamia Nut Ice
  Cream
- Demitasse

Snack
- *Chocolate Fudge
- *Instant Iced Coffee

SUNDAY
Breakfast
- *Cottage Cheese and
  Fruit
- Coffee or Tea

Lunch
- *Macaroni and Cheese
- *Baked Tomato
- *Orange Cooler

Dinner
- *Antipasto
- *Stuffed Steak

- *Stuffed Zippy Zucchini
- *Chocolate Mint Pie
- Diet Soda, Coffee, or Tea

Snack
- *Toasted Almonds
- Diet Soda

LOW FAT MENU PLANS

Dinner
Oven Chicken Breast

LOW FAT MENU PLANS

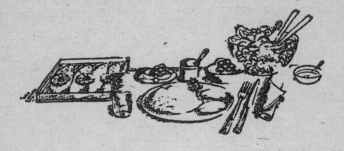

MONDAY
Breakfast
Scrambled Egg Beaters
with Crisp Canadian
Bacon
*Meringue Munchies
Coffee or Tea

Lunch
½ small tomato sliced
Tuna-fish Salad with
Safflower Oil
Mayonnaise
*Rhubarb Snack
Diet Soda

Dinner
*Quick Bouillon
Pickup
*Roast Leg of Lamb
Tossed Salad with Oil
and Vinegar Dressing
*Coffee Foam
Diet Soda, Coffee, or
Tea

Snack
*The "Pop" Pop

TUESDAY
Breakfast
*Tuna and Eggs
Coffee or Tea

Lunch
Crisp Celery Stalks
*Cottage Cheese and
Fruit
*Orange Cooler

Dinner
Clear Chicken Broth
*Oven-Barbecued
Chicken
*Cole Slaw Our Way
(use safflower oil
mayonnaise)
Sugar-free Gelatin
Diet Soda, Coffee, or
Tea

Snack
*Mexican Almonds

WEDNESDAY
Breakfast
*Orange Cooler
*Spanish Omelet
Tea

Lunch
*Fun with Fennel (use
corn oil margarine in
place of butter)
*Glazed Strawberries
Diet Soda, Coffee, or
Tea

Dinner
Celery and Black
Italian Olives
*Scaloppine à la Guido
*Green Bean Salad
*Strawberry-Lemon
Meringue Pie
Demitasse

Snack
  Melon Balls with
    *Strawberry Sauce
  Tea

THURSDAY
Breakfast
  *Fruity Cottage Cheese
  • Salad
  Coffee or Tea

Lunch
  Tossed Salad with
    *Avocado Dressing
    (use safflower oil
    mayonnaise)
  *Tomato Aspic with
    Tuna
  ½ Cantaloupe
  Iced Coffee

Dinner
  *Quick Bouillon
    Pickup
  *Tasty Tender Flank
    Steak
  Sliced Cucumber,
    Green Pepper, and
    Radishes
  *Sherry Dressing (use 1
    cup safflower oil and
    ½ cup olive oil)
  *Blueberry Whip
  Coffee or Tea

Snack
  Sugar-free Gelatin
  *Orange Cooler

FRIDAY
Breakfast
  *Cottage Cheese
    Omelet
  *Meringue Munchies
  Coffee or Tea

Lunch
  *Leftover Veal Salad
  *Cantaloupe and Wine
  Diet Soda

Dinner
  *Italian Garlic Soup
  *Quick Italian Supper
  *Meringue shell filled
    with *Rhubarb-
    Strawberry Jelly
  Coffee or Tea

Snack
  Celery Stuffed with
    Peanut Butter
  Diet Soda or Iced
    Coffee

SATURDAY
Breakfast
  *Orange Cooler
  *Peppers and Eggs
  Coffee or Tea

Lunch
  *Cottage Caesar
  Crisp Canadian Bacon
  *Strawberry Sponge
  Coffee or Tea

Dinner
   Clam Broth
   *Fish Delish (use corn
      oil margarine in
      place of butter)
   Tossed Salad with Oil
      and Vinegar Dressing
   *Meringue Shell filled
      with Fresh Blue-
      berries
   Coffee or Tea

Snack
   Sugar-free Gelatin
      topped with Pecans

SUNDAY
Breakfast
   *Fluffy Jam Omelet
   Dried Beef lightly
      sautéed in 1 teaspoon
      corn oil margarine
   Coffee or Tea

Lunch
   *Tossed Salad with
      Tomato Dressing
   *Pretty Ginger Ale
      Mold
   Iced Tea

Dinner
   Celery and Stuffed
      Olives
   *Salmon à la
      Napolitana
   Sliced Cucumbers with
      *Poppy Seed Dessert
      Dressing
   Melon Balls with
      *Strawberry Sauce
   Coffee or Tea

Snack
   *The "Pop" Pop
   Salted Walnuts

BUFFET MENUS

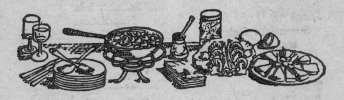

BRUNCH BUFFET
*Orange Cooler
*Ham and Asparagus
  Rolls in Sauce
*Shrimp Curry with
  Eggs
Coffee or Tea
*Island Cottage Cheese
*Meringue Shell filled
  with *Blueberry-
  Raspberry Jam
Chablis with Crushed
  Strawberries Afloat

LUNCHEON BUFFET
Hors d'oeuvres
  *Taste Delight
    Pancakes
  *Mushroom Sauce Dip
  *Heavenly Wings

Appetizer
  *Cantaloupe and Wine

Entrées
  *Fresh Spring Salmon
    Mousse
  *Baked Spinach
  *Mushroom Salad

Desserts
  *Strawberry-Lemon
    Meringue Pie
  *Coconut Drops

Beverage
  Coffee or Tea

DINNER BUFFET
Hors d'oeuvres
  Melon Balls
  Hard Cheese Platter

Entrées
  *Beef Stroganoff
  *Coq au Vin
  *Ratatouille
  Tossed Greens with
    *Dressing of the
    House

Wine
  Dry Chablis

Desserts
  *Meringue Shell filled
    with *Glazed
    Strawberries
  *Coconut Snowflakes
  *Chocolate Cream
    Debbie

Snack
  *Toasted Almonds

Beverage
  Coffee or Tea

SIT-DOWN DINNER
Hors d'oeuvres
  *Meatballs in Dill
  *Deviled-Salmon Eggs
  *Stuffed Mushrooms

Soup
  *Stracciatella

Salad—Appetizer
  *Antipasto

Pasta
  *Manicotti

Entrée
  *Veal Scallopini at Its
    Best

Wine
  Dry Chianti

Desserts
  *Zabaglione with
    *Italian Sponge Cake

Beverage
  Demitasse or
    *Cappuccino

APPETIZERS AND SNACKS

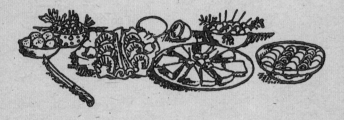

Chipped Beef Balls

12 balls

8 ounces cream cheese,
    at room temperature
1/4 teaspoon sage
1/4 teaspoon onion juice
1/4 teaspoon Worcester-
    shire sauce*

dash of lemon juice
dash of Tabasco sauce
5 ounces chipped or
    dried beef, chopped

Mix together all ingredients except chipped beef.

Chill for at least 1 hour.

Shape into small balls and roll in chipped beef. Refrigerate. Serve on toothpicks.

Total Grams   4.8
Grams per serving   .4

* We have used Lea & Perrins because it is the lowest in carbohydrate grams—1 tablespoon has a trace.

Serve on garnished tray.

Swedish Meatballs

30 meatballs

1/4 cup heavy cream
1/4 cup water
1/4 cup fried pork rinds,*
    crushed
1/2 pound ground round
    beef
1/4 pound ground pork
1/4 pound ground veal
    caraway seeds

1 large onion, chopped
    fine
3 tablespoons butter
2 teaspoons seasoned
    salt*
1/2 recipe Cream Sauce
    (see Index)
    nutmeg

* We have used the products Baken-ets and Krazy Mixed-Up Salt both for taste and because they contain no sugar.

Mix heavy cream and water together. Add pork rinds and allow to soak. Combine beef, pork, and veal.

Sauté onion in 1 tablespoon butter until light brown.

Mix cream mixture, meat, and onion together. Season with salt. Shape into small balls, and brown in 2 tablespoons butter.

Remove balls to chafing dish and keep warm.

Make cream sauce and pour over meatballs. Garnish with nutmeg and caraway seeds.

Total Grams 16.3
Grams per meatball .5

Satisfies the most gourmet taste!

Nutty Cocktail Balls

22 balls

1 pound ground round steak	½ cup chopped walnuts
3 tablespoons sour cream	1 clove garlic, minced
2 teaspoons diced onion	2 teaspoons seasoned salt
	3 tablespoons butter

Mix first 6 ingredients together thoroughly. Shape into 1-inch round balls.

Brown in butter. Serve on toothpicks.

Total Grams 22.4
Grams per ball 1.0

Only one at a time!

Meatballs in Dill

24 meatballs

¼ cup grated Parmesan
  cheese
1½ pounds ground beef
2 eggs, beaten
½ cup chopped onions

1 small clove garlic,
  minced
½ teaspoon nutmeg
½ teaspoon paprika
salt and pepper to taste

3 tablespoons butter

Mix all ingredients except butter in large bowl. Shape into small meatballs. Melt butter in skillet. Brown balls in butter. Place in baking dish.

Sauce
1 teaspoon tomato sauce*
1 teaspoon beef bouillon (dry) in ½ cup broth
1 egg yolk, beaten
½ pint sour cream
2 tablespoons dillseed

Stir tomato sauce and beef bouillon together in saucepan. Add egg yolk. Stir over low flame for 5 minutes. Cool.

Add sour cream and dillseed. Stir well. Pour sauce over meatballs. Bake in 300° oven for 20 minutes.

Total Grams   11.3
Grams per meatball   .5

* We have made these recipes and gram counts with Hunt's tomato sauce because it has a somewhat lower carbohydrate gram count than some tomato sauces.

Entertaining on a diet!

Antipasto

12 servings

1 cup tarragon vinegar
(or any white vinegar)
2 cups olive oil
5 cloves garlic, crushed
1 tablespoon oregano
1½ pounds green olives
½ pound black olives
1 stalk celery, chopped
1 hot red pepper,
chopped

1 small onion, chopped
½ pound Provolone
cheese, diced
½ pound prosciutto, diced
¼ pound Italian salami,
diced
1 7-ounce can tuna fish
lettuce

Mix vinegar, oil, garlic, and oregano together. Add olives, celery, pepper, and onion. Refrigerate overnight. Mix frequently.

Before serving, add Provolone, prosciutto, salami, and tuna fish. Toss well. Serve on lettuce leaves.

Total Grams   48.8
Grams per serving   4.1

No one will believe you're on a diet!

Sweet Cheese Snack

18 snacks

4 ounces cream cheese, at room temperature
2 eggs, separated
1 tablespoon white sugar substitute

Preheat oven to 350°.

Cream the cheese with egg yolks until smooth. Add sugar substitute. Beat egg whites until stiff, but not dry. Fold cheese mixture into stiff whites. Be careful not to break down egg whites.

Grease * cookie sheet. Drop mixture by teaspoonfuls onto cookie sheet and bake in 350° oven for 10 minutes.

Total Grams 5.2
Grams per snack .3

* We use Pam.

A happy combination—sweet and cheesy!

Heavenly Wings

Hors d'oeuvres for 6

1½ pounds chicken wings
1 cup soy protein seasoning
2 tablespoon-equivalents sugar substitute*
¼ cup white wine

2 cloves garlic, mashed
¼ cup oil
1 teaspoon monosodium glutamate
½ teaspoon ground ginger

Preheat oven to 325°.

Wash wings and pat dry. Cut into pieces at joints. Discard wing tips. Combine remaining ingredients for sauce.

Spread wings in shallow baking dish. Do not overlap. Pour sauce over wings. Marinate for 16 hours in refrigerator.

Bake in marinade in 325° oven for 1½ hours.

Total Grams 17.4
Grams per serving 3.0

* A teaspoon-equivalent is the manufacturer's suggestion of how much sugar substitute is equivalent to one teaspoon of sugar.

Finger-licking good!

Cucumbers in Sour Cream

4 servings

1 large cucumber, thinly sliced
½ teaspoon salt
½ cup sour cream
¼ teaspoon-equivalent sugar substitute
1 tablespoon vinegar
½ teaspoon dill

In shallow bowl place cucumber, and sprinkle with salt.

Allow to set for ½ hour. Drain.

Add remaining ingredients. Mix well. Chill.

Total Grams 13.5
Grams per person 3.3

Cheese Balls

12 balls

3 tablespoons butter, softened
4 ounces cream cheese, at room temperature
2 teaspoons heavy cream
⅛ teaspoon seasoned salt
½ cup chopped walnuts

Cream butter, cream cheese, heavy cream, and salt together. Shape into small balls.

Roll in walnuts.

Refrigerate on waxed paper until firm.

Total Grams 22.6
Grams per serving 1.9

Bite-size good!

Fun with Fennel

24 balls

½ pound pot cheese
4 tablespoons fennel seeds
4 tablespoons butter, melted
1 tablespoon-equivalent sugar substitute
1 egg, beaten

Preheat oven to 350°.

Combine all ingredients. Shape into balls. Grease cookie sheet. Place balls on sheet.

Bake for 15 minutes.

Served hot or cold.

Total Grams 8.0

Snick-snacks!

Swiss Snack

1 serving

¼ lb. Swiss cheese, cut into 8 cubes
4 slices bacon
oil

Wrap each cube of cheese in ½ slice bacon. Fry in very hot deep oil for 30 seconds.

Total Grams 4.1

You'll yodel its praises!

Cottage Cheese Dip

1 cup cottage cheese	½ teaspoon caraway seed
1 teaspoon grated onion	½ teaspoon sage
3 tablespoons heavy cream	½ teaspoon celery salt
	1 tablespoon lemon juice

Combine cottage cheese, onion, heavy cream, caraway seed, sage, and celery salt. Mix well. Stir in lemon juice.

Serve with fried pork rinds.

Total Grams 10.8

For "don't-remind-me-I'm-on-a-diet" nibblers!

Cheese It

28 balls

¼ cup blue cheese
½ cup cream cheese
½ pound sliced Swiss cheese

Cream blue cheese and cream cheese together. Spread on Swiss cheese slices. Roll them up and hold together with toothpicks. Refrigerate until firm. Slice into rounds.

Total Grams 6.7
Gram per ball .24

Three cheeses are better than one!

Cottage Cheese Slices

20 slices

1 cup cottage cheese
¼ cup crumbled blue
cheese
5 stuffed olives, chopped
2 tablespoons chopped
pimento

1 tablespoon minced
green pepper
1 tablespoon chopped
parsley
3 tablespoons butter
½ teaspoon paprika

Blend cheeses together well.

Add remaining ingredients. Form into log about 2 inches in diameter.

Wrap in wax paper. Chill. Slice.

Total Grams   14.5
Grams per slice   .7

Snack on a slice!

Sour Cream Clam Dip

1 cup sour cream
1 7½-ounce can minced
clams, drained
2 teaspoons clam juice
(from can)
1 tablespoon grated
onion

1 teaspoon celery seed
¼ cup mayonnaise
1 tablespoon lemon
juice
seasoned salt to taste
(or salt and pepper)

Mix all ingredients together well.

Refrigerate for at least 1 hour. Serve with fried pork rinds.

Total Grams   16.4

Use as a dip for fresh vegetables and count your grams.

Shrimp Appetizers

12 appetizers

- 12 fresh shrimp, cooked
- 4 drops Tabasco sauce
- 2 tablespoons lemon juice
- 1 teaspoon Worcestershire sauce
  salt to taste
- 6 strips bacon

Preheat oven to 425°.

Place shrimp in bowl and add Tabasco sauce, lemon juice, Worcestershire sauce, and salt. Stir until shrimp are well coated.

Cut bacon strips in half. Wrap each shrimp with half a bacon strip and secure with toothpick.

Place in oven in broiler pan. Bake, not broil, until bacon is crisp.

Total Grams 10.8
Grams per shrimp .8

Crunchy shrimp!

Skewered Shrimp and Bacon

18 appetizers

- 18 shelled and deveined shrimp
- 2 tablespoons olive oil
- 1 tablespoon lemon juice
  salt and pepper
  paprika
- 18 strips bacon

Marinate shrimp in oil, lemon juice, and seasonings for several hours. Wrap each shrimp in bacon strip and secure with wet toothpick or small skewer.

Broil, turning often, until bacon is crisp and shrimp are bright pink.

Total Grams 7.6
Grams per shrimp 4.0

Betcha can't eat just one!

Shrimp and Mushroom Appetizer

6 servings

1 pound firm white mushrooms	⅛ teaspoon minced garlic
¼ cup olive oil	1 pound cleaned shrimp, cooked
½ teaspoon lemon juice	1¼ teaspoons salt
⅛ teaspoon freshly ground black pepper	2 tablespoons minced parsley

Wash and dry mushrooms. Remove stems and use for another purpose. Slice caps paper thin; add oil, lemon juice, pepper, and garlic to caps. Marinate in refrigerator for 2 hours, mixing frequently.

Thirty minutes before serving, mix in shrimp and salt. Season to taste. Sprinkle with parsley.

Total Grams 21.8
Grams per serving 3.6

Total taste!

Salami and Parmesan

8 appetizers

½ pound salami, cut into eight cubes
2 eggs, beaten
4 tablespoons grated Parmesan cheese
   oil

Dip salami into beaten eggs and then into Parmesan cheese. Repeat. Fry in deep hot oil for 30 seconds.

Total Grams 4.0

A different delicious combo!

Pickled Seafood

24 pieces

1 pound fresh fillets of
   herring, trout,
   salmon, halibut, or
   whiting
1 medium onion
¾ cup tarragon vinegar

½ cup water
¼ teaspoon-equivalent
   sugar substitute
1 tablespoon whole
   mixed pickling spice
1 teaspoon salt

Clean and cut fillets into 1-inch pieces.

Slice onion and place fish and onion in layers in crock, widemouth quart jar, or serving dish with cover.

Combine remaining ingredients and bring to boil. Simmer for 10 minutes. Cool until lukewarm.

Pour over fish.

Before serving, cover and place in refrigerator for at least 24 hours. This will keep for several weeks.

Total Grams 23.4
Grams per serving .1

Crabmeat Balls for a Crowd

30 balls

2 tablespoons butter	1 egg
2 tablespoons onion	2 tablespoons cream
1 clove garlic	2 teaspoons curry powder
½ cup grated coconut (unsweetened)	1 teaspoon salt
	½ cup fried pork rinds
2 cups crabmeat (fresh or canned)	½ cup oil

Melt 2 tablespoons butter in skillet. Add onion and garlic. Sauté until light brown. Remove onion and garlic, and set aside.

Add coconut to skillet and sauté until light brown.

Combine crabmeat, egg, cream, curry powder, and salt. Add onion and garlic mixture and coconut. Mix well.

Shape into 1-inch balls. Roll in pork rinds. Heat oil in skillet. Brown crabmeat balls in hot oil. Drain thoroughly on absorbent paper. Serve on toothpicks.

Total Grams   23.8

Be sure to make plenty!

To Prepare Eggs for Stuffing

Gently boil eggs for 15 minutes. Turn often to help keep yolks in center. Run eggs under cold water and remove shells. Slice eggs in half lengthwise. Flatten bottom of egg whites by cutting a small slice off bottom side. Remove yolks and prepare stuffing (see below). Pile filling into egg whites. Refrigerate for at least ½ hour.

Stuffed Eggs (Greek Style)

6 servings

24 Greek olives, pitted
6 hard-cooked eggs
2 tablespoons soft butter
seasoned salt

Purée pitted olives in blender.

Cut eggs in half lengthwise and mash yolks until fine.

Combine olives, yolks, butter, and salt until a smooth paste is formed.

Fill egg whites with mixtures.

Total Grams 6.6

You could stuff yourself—but watch that gram count!

Ham and Egg Balls

10 balls

3 eggs, hard-cooked and
shelled
1 teaspoon minced chives
2 tablespoons
mayonnaise

pinch of paprika
salt to taste
¼ teaspoon white horse-
radish
¼ pound boiled ham

Separate yolks and whites of eggs. Mash yolks with fork. Add chives, mayonnaise, paprika, and salt. Put egg whites in blender with horseradish and ham. Blend until smooth.

Mix two mixtures together. Shape into 1-inch balls.
Refrigerate.

Total Grams 2.2
Grams per ball .2

Easy and make ahead!

Pâté in Aspic

8 servings

8 ounces cream cheese
2 tablespoons Worcestershire sauce
1 2½-ounce can pâté
2½ cups beef broth
2 envelopes unflavored gelatin

Cream cream cheese, 1 tablespoon Worcestershire
sauce, and pâté together. Refrigerate.

Place broth, gelatin, and 1 tablespoon Worcestershire
sauce in saucepan. Stir until it begins to boil.

Place ½ cup gelatin mixture in bottom of 3½ cup
mold. Refrigerate until set.

Remove cheese mixture from refrigerator and form
into ball. Place in center of mold.

Pouring remaining 2 cups gelatin mixture around pâté
ball.

Return to refrigerator until set. Unmold on plate.

Total Grams 13.4
Grams per serving 1.7

For a gourmet taste—and look.

Spiced Black Olives

24 olives

2 7½-ounce cans pitted jumbo black olives, drained
2 teaspoons crushed red pepper
2 teaspoons pickling spice
2 small cloves garlic, crushed
¼ cup red wine vinegar
¼ cup olive or salad oil

Combine all ingredients in container with tight-fitting lid. Shake gently to mix. Refrigerate for several days. Shake occasionally. Drain before serving. These can be stored several weeks in refrigerator.

Total Grams 11.1
Grams per olive .5

Something extra.

Buttered Radishes

24 radishes

12 perfect radishes with stems
¼ pound lightly salted butter, at room temperature
1 tablespoon cream cheese

¼ teaspoon dry mustard
¼ teaspoon lemon juice
¼ teaspoon onion juice
¼ teaspoon caraway seeds
dash of Tabasco sauce
nutmeg

Cut radishes in half lengthwise.

Cream butter with cream cheese. Blend in mustard, lemon juice, onion juice, caraway seeds, and Tabasco sauce. Chill until firm enough to be pushed through pastry tube. Squeeze onto surface of each radish half. Chill. Sprinkle with nutmeg.

Total Grams   5.4
Grams per radish   .23

Pretties up your hors d'oeuvres platter!

Deviled-Salmon Eggs

12 egg halves

6 hard-cooked eggs	½ teaspoon lemon juice
3 tablespoons mayonnaise	1 teaspoon prepared mustard
½ cup boned and flaked salmon, canned or smoked	1 teaspoon Worcester-shire sauce
	½ teaspoon salt

dash of pepper

Cut eggs in half lengthwise. Remove yolks, reserving whites.

Mash yolks and mayonnaise together until smooth. Add remaining ingredients (reserve enough salmon for garnish) and mix well.

Spoon mixture into egg whites.

Garnish with pieces of salmon.

Total Grams 4.0
Grams per serving   Trace

Devilishly good!

Stuffed Mushrooms

6 servings

½ pound large white
    mushrooms
4 tablespoons butter
⅛ cup chopped onion
1 tablespoon chicken fat
    (or butter)
¼ pound chicken livers
    (½ cup)

3 tablespoons cream
    cheese
salt and pepper to taste
1 egg, hard-cooked and
    chopped

Remove stems from mushrooms. Chop stems. Heat butter in skillet. Sauté mushroom caps. Remove from pan and set aside. Sauté onion and mushroom stems in butter until onion is light brown. Remove from pan. Add chicken fat to pan and brown chicken livers. Cool livers. Chop them.

Cream together cream cheese with liver, mushrooms, and onion. Add salt and pepper.

Stuff mixture into mushroom caps, garnish with chopped eggs, and serve.

Total Grams 16.6
Grams per serving 2.8

It's what's inside that makes the difference!

Mexican Almonds

320 almonds in a pound

1 pound blanched almonds
2 tablespoons oil
¼ teaspoon chili powder
1 teaspoon salt
dash of pepper

Sauté almonds in oil for about 5 minutes. Drain on paper towels. Add seasonings.

Total Grams 88.5

Bueno! Bueno! Bueno!

Cheddar Olives

28 olives

28 large pimento-stuffed green olives
2 cups (1 pound) grated sharp Cheddar cheese
½ pound sliced bacon

Halve large stuffed olives lengthwise. Remove pimentos and chop fine. Blend cheese with pimentos.

Stuff olive halves with this mixture. Press halves together.

Cut bacon slices in half. Wrap each olive in ½ slice bacon. Secure with toothpick.

Broil 4 to 5 minutes on each side or until bacon is crisp.

Total Grams 14.7
Grams per serving .5

Olives and Cheddar were never better!

Rhubarb Snack

1 serving

½ cup cottage cheese
2 tablespoons Rhubarb-Strawberry Jelly (see Index)

Mix together.

Total Grams 5.3

A sweet surprise!

Toasted Almonds

About 320 almonds in a pound

1 pound blanched whole almonds
½ cup vegetable oil
  seasoned salt to taste

Preheat oven to 350°.

Put almonds in large baking dish. Sprinkle with oil and salt. All almonds should be coated with oil.

Bake in 350° oven until almonds turn light brown. Shake pan occasionally.

Total Grams 88.5

For TV watchers!

SOUPS

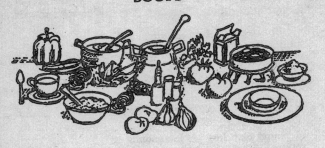

Quick Bouillon Pickup

1 serving

1 cup hot bouillon
1 egg
    dash of Tabasco sauce
    dash of salt

Blend egg in electric blender until light and foamy. Add bouillon slowly. Blend in Tabasco sauce and salt.

Serve hot in mug.

Total Grams   1.6

Try it—you'll love it!

Creamy Dumplings for Soup

4 servings

1 tablespoon soft butter
1 egg plus 1 yolk
½ cup heavy cream
½ teaspoon seasoned salt
    pinch of nutmeg
    chicken broth

Spray top of double boiler with grease substitute. Rub with butter.

Beat eggs, heavy cream, salt, and nutmeg together with fork. Pour into top of double boiler.

Cook over hot (not boiling) water for 45 minutes, or until set and firm. Turn out onto waxed paper and cool. Slice into cubes. Add to clear hot broth. Serve immediately.

> Total Grams 5.3
> Grams per serving 1.3

Simply delicious!

Cottage Cheese in Cream Soup

8 servings

1 onion, chopped fine
1 stalk celery, chopped
2 green peppers, chopped
3 tablespoons butter
1½ teaspoons salt
¼ teaspoon fresh white pepper
½ teaspoon paprika

3 cups water
½ pound cottage cheese (1 cup)
3 cups heavy cream (1½ pints)
2 sprigs parsley, minced
3 strips bacon, fried crisp

Sauté onion, celery, and peppers in butter until onion turns golden (10 to 15 minutes).

Add salt, pepper, paprika, and water. Cover and simmer gently for 1 hour.

Add cottage cheese and put mixture in blender. Blend at medium speed until smooth.

Add heavy cream and heat, but do not boil.

Garnish with minced parsley and bacon pieces. Serve hot.

> Total Grams 22.4
> Grams per serving 3.7

Something very different!

Creamy Mushroom Soup

10 servings

½ pound mushrooms, sliced thin
¼ pound butter
1 quart chicken broth
1 quart beef broth
2 tablespoons crushed

toasted sesame seeds (crush in blender)
½ teaspoon seasoned salt
1 cup heavy cream
1 tablespoon minced chives

Sauté mushrooms in half the butter for 5 minutes.

Mix broths; add mushrooms. Melt remaining butter in saucepan. Add crushed sesame seeds. Gradually add some broth, stirring steadily.

Return sesame mixture to balance of broth. Add salt. Cook over low heat for 10 minutes. Stir in heavy cream until well blended.

Serve in cups with garnish of chives.

Total Grams 20.7
Grams per serving 2.1

Oh, that mushroom flavor!

Onion Soup

8 servings

1½ large Bermuda onions, chopped
¼ pound butter
8 cups boiling water
8 beef bouillon cubes
2 tablespoons Worcestershire sauce

2 teaspoons gravy extender*
grated Parmesan cheese

Sauté onions in butter until brown around edges. Add boiling water and beef bouillon.

Add Worcestershire sauce and gravy extender. Stir well. Simmer for ½ hour, stirring occasionally. Pour into soup bowls and sprinkle with Parmesan cheese.

Total Grams 40.1
Grams per serving 5.0

° We have used Gravy Master.

Extra good if refrigerated overnight.

Avocado Cream Soup Barbara

8 servings (½ cup each)

1 medium avocado
2 cups heavy cream
1 cup water
½ teaspoon celery salt
¼ teaspoon seasoned salt

½ small clove garlic, minced
8 slices bacon, cooked crisp

Peel avocado and remove pit. Place in blender with heavy cream, water, celery salt, salt, and garlic. Blend at medium speed for 15 seconds.

Pour into saucepan. Cook over medium heat for 5 minutes, stirring constantly. Do not boil.

Serve warm or cold garnished with crumbled bacon.

Total Grams 29.7
Grams per serving 3.7

An impressive first course!

Senegalese Soup

6 servings

2 onions, chopped
2 stalks celery, chopped
¼ cantaloupe, peeled and chopped
4 tablespoons butter
1 tablespoon curry powder
4 cups broth (can be made from bouillon cubes)

½ teaspoon salt
⅛ teaspoon chili powder
⅛ teaspoon cayenne pepper
1 cup heavy cream
1½ cups chopped cooked chicken
¼ avocado, chopped

Sauté onions, celery, and cantaloupe in butter until onions are golden. Add curry powder. Stir in chicken broth and other seasonings. Simmer for about 5 minutes.

Purée mixture in blender (about half at a time). Chill.

Just before serving, add heavy cream and chicken. Stir well. Spoon into soup bowls and garnish with avocado.

Total Grams 34.8
Grams per serving 5.7

Soup exotica!

Gazpacho

6 servings

¼ teaspoon garlic
powder
1 onion, chopped
4 parsley sprigs
2 tablespoons vinegar
3 tablespoons olive oil
¼ teaspoon cayenne
pepper
¼ teaspoon seasoned salt

1½ cups chicken broth
4 large tomatoes, peeled
2 tablespoons chopped
cucumber
2 tablespoons chopped
green pepper
2 tablespoons crushed
fried pork rinds

Place all ingredients except last 3 in blender. Blend until smooth. Chill overnight.

Serve in chilled bowls. Garnish each with 1 teaspoon cucumber, pepper, and fried pork rinds.

Total Grams   31.7
Grams per serving   5.3

Serve with gusto!

Stracciatella Soup

6 servings

1 pound fresh spinach
or 2 frozen packages
2 tablespoons butter
1¼ teaspoons salt
¼ teaspoon white pepper
⅛ teaspoon nutmeg

4 egg yolks
¼ cup grated Parmesan
cheese
6 cups boiling chicken
broth

Cook spinach for 4 minutes. Drain thoroughly. Purée in electric blender or force through sieve.

Melt butter in saucepan; add spinach, salt, pepper, and nutmeg. Cook over low heat for 2 minutes, stirring constantly.

Beat egg yolks and Parmesan cheese. Pour into boiling broth and mix with fork. Add spinach mixture. Simmer for 5 minutes. Serve hot.

Total Grams 29.8
Grams per serving 5.0

The name is the most complicated thing about it!

Italian Garlic Soup

4 servings

6 large garlic cloves	1 bay leaf
2 quarts boiling water	2 cloves
2 teaspoons seasoned salt	pinch of saffron
¼ teaspoon thyme	4 egg yolks
¼ teaspoon sage	¼ cup olive oil
parsley sprigs	

Chop garlic and place in boiling water. Add salt, thyme, sage, bay leaf, cloves, and saffron. Boil for 30 minutes.

Beat egg yolks with wire whisk. When thick and creamy, add olive oil 1 teaspoon at a time and beat well after each addition.

Add egg yolks to soup and beat with wire whisk.

Garnish with parsley. Serve immediately.

Total Grams 6.0
Grams per serving 1.5

Spicy soup stuff.

Lobster Soup

6 servings

2 cups fresh or canned lobster meat	1 cup water
3 tablespoons butter	½ teaspoon seasoned salt
3 cups heavy cream	¼ teaspoon onion powder
	¼ cup sherry

Cut lobster meat into bite-size pieces. Melt butter in skillet and add lobster. Cook for 5 minutes over low heat.

Separately mix heavy cream with water. Add to skillet, stirring constantly. Do not boil. Add salt and onion powder. Refrigerate overnight.

Reheat. Add sherry. Serve in soup bowls.

Total Grams 25.5
Grams per serving 4.2

For the easy-cooking gourmet!

Creamy Noodles for Soup

4 servings

1 tablespoon soft butter
1 egg plus 1 yolk
½ cup heavy cream
½ teaspoon seasoned salt
pinch of nutmeg
chicken broth

Spray top of double boiler with grease substitute. Rub butter into grease substitute.

Beat eggs, heavy cream, salt, and nutmeg together with fork. Pour mixture into top of double boiler.

Cook over hot (not boiling) water for 45 minutes or until set and firm. Turn out onto waxed paper and cool. Slice into cubes. Add to clear hot broth.

Total Grams 5.3
Grams per serving 1.3

Simply delicious!

Japanese Egg Custard Soup

6 servings

1 cup julienne-cut cooked chicken or diced shrimp
3 water chestnuts, diced
6 mushrooms, diced
2 scallions, chopped

1 tablespoon sherry
4 eggs, beaten
1 teaspoon salt
3 cups beef broth
12 spinach or lettuce leaves

Preheat oven to 300°.

Combine chicken or shrimp, water chestnuts, mushrooms, scallions, and sherry. Divide equally into 6 custard cups.

Beat eggs, salt, and broth together. Pour into custard cups. Cover with spinach or lettuce leaves.

Place in large pan with 3 inches boiling water. Cover pan and bake in 300° oven for 30 minutes or until mixture is set.

Total Grams 26.2
Grams per serving 4.4

EGGS AND CHEESE

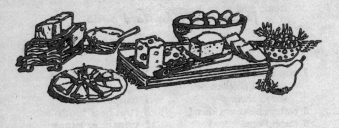

How to Make Omelets

Omelets are made in two basic ways—the plain French omelet and the fluffy soufflé omelet. The difference is in the preparation.

For the plain omelet you beat the whole egg and cook it over direct heat. The fluffy omelet is made by separating the yolks and the whites, beating them separately, folding them together, cooking them over direct heat, and then baking them in the oven.

More about the plain omelet· The right pan is very important. It should be a heavy pan about 2 inches deep, with sloping sides. The size depends on how many eggs you are cooking. Six eggs should be the maximum used in an omelet.

For 2 to 4 eggs use 8-inch pan
For 4 to 6 eggs use 10-inch pan

Always spray the pan with grease substitute before starting your omelet. Heat the pan hot enough to make the butter foamy without burning it. When the pan is hot enough, add the eggs.

Tip the pan to spread the eggs to all sides. Run a spatula around the edge of the pan and tip it again so the uncooked eggs go to the edges.

Repeat this until the center of the omelet is of a jellied consistency. Make a crease in the center of the omelet to make it easier to fold over.

Run the spatula around the edge again to make sure it is not sticking.

Add desired filling and fold the omelet over.

Serve immediately.

Fluffy Jam Omelet

2 servings

1 recipe Basic Fluffy Omelet (see below)
1 teaspoon vanilla extract
2 tablespoons Blueberry-Raspberry Jam (see Index)

Make Basic Fluffy Omelet, except when beating egg yolks, add vanilla extract.

Just before folding, spread omelet with jam. Fold. Serve immediately.

Total Grams 12.8
Grams per serving 6.4

Light and luscious!

Basic Fluffy Omelet

2 servings

4 eggs, separated, and at room temperature
½ teaspoon baking powder
½ teaspoon salt
2 tablespoons heavy cream
2 tablespoons water
1 tablespoon butter

Preheat oven to 300°.

Beat egg whites, baking powder, and salt together until egg whites are stiff.

Beat egg yolks with heavy cream and water. Fold yolk mixture into whites, being very careful not to break down whites.

Spray skillet with grease substitute and melt butter. Pour in eggs. Cook over low heat for about 12 minutes, or until brown on bottom.

Place in oven until top is set. Fold omelet in half and serve at once.

> Total Grams   4.4
> Grams per serving   2.2

Getting down to delicious basics!

Cheese Omelet

2 servings

4 eggs
½ cup grated Cheddar cheese
1 tablespoon chopped parsley

Follow recipe for Basic Fluffy Omelet (see Index). Before folding omelet over, add grated Cheddar cheese and chopped parsley.

After folding omelet over, continue cooking for 2 minutes to be sure cheese is melted.

Serve hot.

> Total Grams   6.0
> Grams per serving   3.0

An easy variation!

Bacon and Onion Omelet

6 servings

9 strips bacon   6 eggs
¼ cup diced onion

Cut bacon into small pieces. Fry in small skillet. Add onion and sauté until all fat melts off bacon. Pour off fat.

Follow recipe for Basic Fluffy Omelet (see Index).

Pour bacon and onion on 1 side of omelet before folding over other side. Fold over and cook 1 minute. Serve immediately.

Total Grams   10.1
Grams per serving   1.7

The only thing better than bacon and eggs is bacon and onion and eggs.

Crabmeat and Mushroom Omelet

6 servings

2 tablespoons butter	½ cup crabmeat
½ cup thinly sliced fresh mushrooms	1 tablespoon sherry
	4 tablespoons cream
1 tablespoon diced onion	6 eggs

Melt butter in skillet. Sauté mushrooms and onion in butter until light brown. Stir in crabmeat. Simmer for 3 minutes. Add sherry and simmer 1 more minute. Add cream.

Follow recipe for Basic Fluffy Omelet (see Index).

Spoon half mixture over half of omelet just before folding, and place remaining mixture over top of omelet after it has been folded.

Total Grams   12.0
Grams per serving   2.0

Distinct flavors, deliciously blended!

Omelet with a Special Taste

4 servings

½ pound chipped beef, in bite-size pieces
½ pound spicy sausage, in bite-size pieces
1 clove garlic, minced
½ cup olive oil
1 teaspoon seasoned salt

1 teaspoon caraway seeds
1 tablespoon tomato paste
2 drops Tabasco sauce
6 eggs, beaten
2 tablespoons grated Parmesan cheese

Preheat oven to 325°.

Sauté beef, sausage, and garlic in olive oil until sausage is well browned. Drain off fat. Add salt, caraway seeds, tomato paste, and Tabasco sauce. Stir well. Cool.

Combine eggs and Parmesan cheese. Spoon meat mixture into baking dish and cover with eggs. Bake in 325° oven for 45 minutes or until set.

Total Grams 11.0
Grams per serving .3

Eggs Florentine

6 servings

2 cups cooked fresh spinach or 1 package frozen spinach
6 eggs
salt to taste
1 recipe Cheese Sauce (see Index)

Preheat oven to 350°.

Cook spinach. Drain well. Chop fine.

Place hot spinach in shallow baking dish.

Make hole for each egg in spinach. Break egg into each hole. Sprinkle with salt.

Prepare cheese sauce. Pour over eggs and spinach.

Bake in moderate 350° oven for 25 minutes.

Total Grams 35.6
Grams per serving 6.0

Cheese and Onion Pie

8 servings

1 large onion
2 tablespoons butter
1½ cups grated Cheddar
    cheese

1 cup heavy cream
1 egg plus 2 yolks
½ teaspoon seasoned salt
pinch of paprika

Preheat oven to 400°.

Sauté onion in butter.

Place half of cheese in 9-inch pie pan sprayed with grease substitute.

Top with ½ sautéed onion. Repeat layers of cheese and onion.

Combine heavy cream, eggs, salt, and paprika to make a sauce. Pour over cheese and onion.

Bake in 400° oven for 15 minutes. Lower heat to 325° and bake for ½ hour more.

Total Grams 31.7
Grams per serving 4.0

Easy, inexpensive—and delicious!

Cheese Soufflé

8 servings for Hors d'oeuvres
4 servings for Main Course

3 tablespoons butter	½ cup grated Swiss Gruyère cheese
1 tablespoon soya powder	⅓ cup grated Parmesan cheese
1 cup heavy cream, scalded	½ ripe Camembert cheese
¼ cup water	2 tablespoons sour cream
½ teaspoon seasoned salt dash of cayenne pepper	2 tablespoons dry sherry
1 teaspoon Dijon mustard	4 egg yolks
½ teaspoon dry mustard	6 egg whites, at room temperature

Preheat oven to 375°.

Prepare soufflé dish by wrapping a 3-inch piece of waxed paper around the outside top of your dish. Tie with string to hold in place. Brush inside of dish and waxed paper with melted butter or margarine.

Melt butter over medium heat. Remove from heat and beat with wire whisk. Add soya. Beat until smooth. Add heavy cream and water, which have been scalded together in separate pot.

Add salt, pepper, mustards, and cheeses (only ½ Parmesan). Beat until smooth. Add sour cream and sherry. Mix. Add 1 egg yolk at a time and beat well. Set aside. Beat egg whites until stiff but not dry.

Fold in cheese mixture with gentle blending motion. Try not to break down egg whites.

Pour into soufflé dish and sprinkle with remaining Parmesan cheese. Bake in 375° oven for about 1 hour, or until brown and hard to the touch.

Serve immediately.

Grams per serving Hors d'oeuvres 2.8
Grams per serving Main Course 5.7

Delicious and worth a little extra time and effort.

Egg Foo Yung

6 servings

2 onions, chopped fine
2 green peppers, chopped
6 slices ham, chopped
1 16-ounce can bean
  sprouts

6 eggs, beaten
  salt and pepper to taste
3 tablespoons peanut oil

Beat first 6 ingredients together.

Heat oil in skillet. Drop mixture into oil by table-spoonfuls. Brown on both sides. Serve with Mustard Sauce (see Index).

Total Grams 36.7
Grams per serving 6.1

For those who love their eggs the Chinese way!

Mushrooms, Onions, and Eggs

3 servings

½ pound mushrooms, sliced
1 small onion, chopped
4 tablespoons butter
  seasoned salt to taste
6 eggs
2 tablespoons heavy cream

Sauté mushrooms and onion in butter until well browned. Add salt.

Beat eggs with heavy cream. Pour over mushroom mixture and stir until eggs are cooked (about 4 stirs). Serve immediately.

Total Grams 18.1
Grams per serving 6.0

To dress up your eggs!

Taste Delight Pancakes

2 servings

½ pound ground beef
3 egg yolks, lightly beaten
1 teaspoon lemon juice
1 tablespoon grated onion
½ teaspoon celery seed

½ teaspoon dry mustard
¼ teaspoon baking powder
½ teaspoon salt
dash of pepper
3 egg whites

oil

Mix first 9 ingredients well.

Beat egg whites stiff. Fold meat mixture into beaten egg whites.

Lightly oil hot griddle or skillet. Drop mixture on griddle by tablespoonfuls. Lift edge of pancake to see if it is browned and puffy. Turn with spatula and brown other side.

Good served with or without sauce. For a delicious treat, serve with Mushroom Sauce (see Index).

Total Grams 2.8
Grams per serving 1.4

Just what the name implies!

Eggs and Swiss Cheese

2 servings

4 ounces Swiss cheese slices	⅛ teaspoon caraway seeds
4 eggs	½ teaspoon seasoned salt
⅛ teaspoon nutmeg	2 tablespoons butter
	¼ cup heavy cream
cayenne pepper	

Preheat oven to 400°.

Lay half of Swiss cheese slices in bottom of baking dish.

Beat eggs. Add nutmeg, caraway seeds, and salt to eggs. Pour into baking dish. Add remaining cheese. Dot with butter. Pour heavy cream into baking dish. Dust with pepper. Bake in 400° oven for 15 minutes until set.

Total Grams 9.4
Grams per serving 4.7

Scrambled Eggs in Cheese Sauce with Sausages

6 servings

12 link sausages	¾ cup cream
1 3-ounce package cream cheese	¼ cup water
	1 teaspoon seasoned salt
1 tablespoon butter	2 teaspoons parsley
8 eggs, beaten	

Sauté sausages in skillet until brown. Drain.

In double boiler over simmering (not boiling) water, heat cream cheese and butter. Add cream, water, salt and parsley.

Stir in beaten eggs with fork. Cook until eggs have thickened.

Total Grams   15.9
Grams per serving   2.6

Breakfast, noon, or nighttime too!

Cheese Pancakes

6 servings

1 cup cottage cheese
6 eggs
3 tablespoons soya powder
3 tablespoons butter, melted
1 teaspoon seasoned salt
  oil

Put all ingredients except oil in blender. Blend until smooth. Heat oiled griddle until very hot. Drop batter by tablespoonfuls onto griddle. Brown on both sides.

Serve with Spicy Blueberry Jam (see Index).

Total Grams   22.2
Grams per serving   3.5

Eat them at the beginning or end of the day!

MEAT

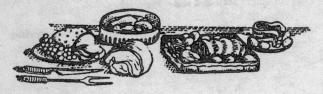

Ham and Egg Fritters

12 fritters

¼ cup soya powder
3 ounces water
1 egg, slightly beaten
¼ teaspoon baking
    powder
¼ teaspoon seasoned salt

3 hard-cooked eggs
2 slices boiled ham
2 tablespoons olive oil
½ recipe Mustard Sauce
    (see Index)

Place soya powder in bowl. Add water gradually, and beat until well blended. Stir in beaten egg, baking powder, and salt.

Chop hard-cooked eggs with ham. Add to soya batter and mix well.

Heat olive oil in heavy skillet until it begins to smoke. Drop mixture by tablespoonfuls into hot oil. Brown on one side and turn. Remove from oil and drain well on absorbent paper.

Serve immediately with mustard sauce, or refrigerate, and warm later on cookie sheet in 350° oven for 10 minutes.

Total Grams   26.2
Grams per fritter   2.2

An updated old-fashioned favorite!

Baked Ham Soufflé

4 servings

2 tablespoons butter,
    melted
1 cup heavy cream,
    scalded

4 egg yolks
2 cups finely chopped ham
    seasoned salt
    nutmeg

6 egg whites

Preheat oven to 350°.

Prepare soufflé dish (see Index).

In top of double boiler combine melted butter and scalded heavy cream. Add egg yolks and beat with rotary beater for about 5 minutes or until mixture thickens. Add ham. Cool. Season with salt and nutmeg.

In large bowl beat egg whites until stiff, but not dry. Pour cool mixture over stiff egg whites and gently fold ingredients together in, under, and over mixture. Do not break down egg whites.

Pour into buttered soufflé dish and cook in 350° oven for 25 minutes, or until firm on top.

Total Grams   9.1
Grams per serving   2.3

Heavenly light!

Ham and Asparagus Rolls in Sauce

12 rolls

24 stalks asparagus, cooked (about 1 pound)
12 slices baked or boiled ham

Cheese Sauce
¾ cup cream
⅓ cup water
¾ pound or 1½ cups diced Cheddar cheese
1 teaspoon mustard
1 teaspoon salt
½ teaspoon paprika

Preheat oven to 350°.

Place 2 stalks cooked asparagus on each ham slice lengthwise. Roll slices and secure with toothpicks.

Place in baking dish. Set aside.

In double boiler combine ingredients for cheese sauce. Simmer slowly. Stir constantly until smooth.

Pour cheese sauce over ham rolls.

Bake, covered, in 350° oven for 15 to 20 minutes until thoroughly heated.

Total Grams 25.2
Grams per serving 2.1

Cook carefully!

Hungarian Ham Pancakes

2 servings

1 recipe Pasta (see Index)

Ham Filling
½ pound boiled ham, chopped
1 egg yolk
½ cup sour cream
¼ teaspoon paprika
1 teaspoon butter

Preheat oven to 350°.

Combine all ingredients except butter.

Lightly oil baking dish. Place 1 heaping tablespoon ham filling on top of pancake. Repeat. Place butter on last pancake.

Bake in 350° oven for about 20 to 25 minutes. Cut in half to serve.

Total Grams 6.0
Grams per serving 3.0

A Pork Chop Meal

6 servings

12 pork chops
 salt and pepper to
  taste
2 tablespoons vegetable
  oil
2 tablespoons olive oil
1 onion, chopped
1 clove garlic, minced

1 pound mushrooms,
  sliced
1½ cups hot chicken broth
½ cup dry red wine
1 bay leaf
¼ cup sour cream
  (optional)

Preheat oven to 350°.

Sprinkle pork chops with salt and pepper. Brown chops in vegetable oil over high heat. Remove and keep warm.

Add olive oil to pan. Sauté onion, garlic, and mushrooms in olive oil until onion is golden. Pour in chicken broth, wine, and add bay leaf. Bring mixture to boil and cook for about 3 minutes.

Arrange 6 pork chops in casserole. Top with half the vegetables from mixture (remove them with slotted spoon). Put another layer of pork chops on top and pour over remaining mixture. Cover casserole tightly and bake in 350° oven for 1½ hours.

If desired, sour cream may be added to mixture when served.

Total Grams 36.9
Grams per serving 6.2

A marvelous main dish!

Breaded Veal Cutlets in Wine Sauce

6 servings

½ cup grated Parmesan cheese	2 eggs, beaten
¼ teaspoon garlic powder	4 tablespoons butter
¼ teaspoon oregano	½ cup chicken broth
6 veal cutlets	4 tablespoons dry white wine

6 lemon slices

Mix cheese with garlic powder and oregano. Dip veal cutlets into cheese, then into egg, and back into cheese. Make sure you cover veal each time.

Melt butter in skillet, and brown veal on both sides. Take veal from pan and keep warm. Pour broth and wine into skillet. Boil for about 1 minute. Pour liquid over warm veal. Garnish with lemon slices.

Total Grams 4.6
Grams per serving .8

If you like cheese, this egg-cheese breading may be used in almost any recipe for veal or chicken.

Roast Veal

6 servings

4- or 5-pound veal roast (leg, loin, rump, shoulder, or breast)	3 tablespoons oil
1 clove garlic, minced	4 tablespoons chopped onion
5 or 6 anchovies (optional)	2 celery stalks, diced
	½ cup white wine or broth

Preheat oven to 325°.

Have the butcher bone and tie meat, and lard it by placing salt pork on it.

Cut a few incisions in veal and insert minced garlic and a few anchovies.

In roasting pan with cover, heat oil and brown veal. Add onion, celery, and wine to pan. Place in 325° oven, covered, and baste occasionally. Allow 30 minutes a pound.

Remove veal from pan, and let it set for 10 minutes for easier carving.

Remove vegetables from pan juices, skim off excess fat, and pour pan juices over veal.

Serve cold sliced the next day with Vinaigrette Cream Dressing (see Index) or Dressing of the House (see Index).

Total Grams 16
Grams per serving 2.4

Veal and Avocado

4 servings

1½ pounds veal cutlet	salt to taste
4 tablespoons butter	1 small can shrimp
½ cup chicken broth	½ medium avocado,
4 or 5 drops lemon juice	sliced
2 teaspoons parsley	

Cut meat in 2 or 3 places around edges to prevent curling. Place in skillet and sauté in 3 tablespoons butter until well browned. Remove to warm dish.

Pour broth in skillet. Boil, stirring well, and reduce liquid to half. Add lemon juice, parsley, and salt to broth.

Sauté shrimp in 1 tablespoon butter for about 4 or 5 minutes, stirring constantly. Spoon broth over veal. Top with shrimp.

Garnish with thin slices of avocado.

Total Grams 13.3
Grams per serving 3.3

Scaloppine à la Guido

6 servings

2 pounds milk-fed veal, cut for scaloppini
3 tablespoons olive oil
3 tablespoons diced onion
2 cups red Burgundy wine

Pound veal with mallet to be sure all fibers are broken down. It should be thin (about 3 inches in diameter).

Place oil in large skillet. Add onion and sauté until light brown. Push to side of pan.

Add veal and sauté for about 5 minutes on each side.

Add Burgundy. Simmer until sauce turns brown—about 12 minutes.

Total Grams 8.6
Grams per serving 1.3

Veal Scaloppine at Its Best

6 servings

1½ pounds veal cut into scallops ¼-inch thick
seasoned salt to taste
6 tablespoons butter
¼ cup brandy
1 cup chicken broth
¼ cup Chablis
2 tablespoons dry sherry

1 pound mushrooms
2 tomatoes, peeled
1 teaspoon garlic powder
½ cup grated Swiss cheese
¼ cup grated Parmesan cheese

Sprinkle veal with salt. Melt 4 tablespoons butter in skillet. Brown veal in butter.

Heat brandy. Ignite it. Pour over veal. Remove veal from pan and keep warm. Place chicken broth, Chablis, and sherry in pan. Simmer until liquid reduces to half. Put veal back in pan. Simmer for 10 minutes. Keep warm.

Wash and slice mushrooms. Sauté in 2 tablespoons butter until brown. Add peeled tomatoes and garlic powder. Simmer for 5 minutes. Place mushroom mixture in baking dish. Add veal and cover with wine sauce. Sprinkle with grated Swiss and Parmesan cheeses.

Broil until cheese is brown and bubbly. Serve immediately.

Total Grams 40.5
Grams per serving 6.7

*You never would have believed
the best could be so good!*

Hungarian Veal Stew

4 servings

3 strips bacon, diced	2 pounds cubed veal
3 tablespoons butter	½ cup water or stock
1 tablespoon chopped onion	1 cup sour cream
	1 teaspoon salt
½ cup sliced mushrooms	¼ teaspoon paprika

Preheat oven to 250°.

Place bacon, butter, onion, and mushrooms in skillet. Sauté slowly until onion and bacon are lightly brown.

Remove bacon, onion, and mushrooms with slotted spoon. Place in oven-proof baking dish. Leave bacon fat and butter in skillet.

Add veal to fat in skillet. Brown meat on all sides. Remove veal, leaving fat in skillet. Place meat in baking dish. Mix well with bacon mixture.

Place water, sour cream, salt, and paprika in skillet. Heat just to boiling. Pour over meat mixture. Cover dish.

Bake in slow 250° oven for 1 hour, or until veal is tender when pierced with fork.

Total Grams 17.4
Grams per serving 4.3

For hearty appetites!

Roast Pork

6 servings

4- or 5-pound pork roast (loin or shoulder)
1 large clove garlic, minced fine
salt and pepper to taste

Preheat oven to 350°.

Wipe meat with damp cloth. Cut off edges and surplus fat.

Cut a small incision in meat and insert garlic. Sprinkle with salt and pepper.

Place meat fat side up in roasting pan. Roast in 350° oven. Cook for 30 to 45 minutes per pound. The meat should be grayish white.

Total Grams Trace

Country Stew

8 servings

4 tablespoons vegetable oil	2 teaspoons salt
3 pounds stew meat (chuck, round)	½ cup cubed rutabaga
	½ cup diced green pepper
4 tablespoons onion, chopped	½ cup cubed eggplant
	1 cup cubed zucchini
4 cups water	4 tablespoons tomato sauce
3 soup bones	1 cup spinach

Heat oil in large heavy pot. Add meat and brown well on all sides. Push meat to one side of pot, and add onion. Cook for 5 more minutes.

Add water, soup bones, and salt. Simmer for 2 hours.

Add rutabaga and simmer for 15 more minutes.

Add green pepper, eggplant, and zucchini. Simmer for 10 more minutes. Spoon in tomato sauce and spinach, and cook for 7 more minutes.

Total Grams 43.9
Grams per serving 5.4

A favorite with children as well as grown-ups; it takes the chill out of the cold wintry air.

Luscious Lamb

4 servings

8 lamb chops garlic powder	2 tablespoons lemon juice
2 tablespoons butter	2 tablespoons gin
2 tablespoons Worcestershire sauce	1 teaspoon seasoned salt

Rub lamb chops with small amount of garlic powder. Melt butter and add Worcestershire sauce, lemon juice, gin, and salt. Pour liquid over lamb chops. Allow to marinate for 15 minutes. Remove lamb from marinade. Broil to desired doneness.

> Total Grams 2.8
> Grams per serving .7

It's amazing what a little marinade will do.

Lamb Sweet Lamb

4 servings

1 3-pound piece shoulder lamb with all fat cut off

1 teaspoon ground ginger

3 tablespoons soy protein seasoning*

2 teaspoons Worcestershire sauce

1 small green pepper, cored and sliced

½ onion, sliced thin

1 large clove garlic, pierced

1 tablespoon-equivalent brown sugar substitute

¼ recipe Spicy Blueberry Jam (see Index)

Preheat oven to 350°

Remove bone from lamb. Rub lamb with ginger, soy protein seasoning, and Worcestershire sauce. Place in baking pan.

Add pepper, onion, and garlic to pan.

Refrigerate overnight, turning occasionally. Before cooking, bring lamb to room temperature, and remove pepper, onion, and garlic. Sprinkle brown sugar substitute over meat and spread with Spicy Blueberry Jam.

Bake for 1¼ hours in 350° oven.

Total Grams 20.0
Grams per serving 5.0

* We have used Maggi's seasoning because it is lower in carbohydrate than other "soy sauces."

Roast Leg of Lamb

4 servings

4- or 5-pound leg of lamb
1 large clove garlic, minced
4 tablespoons prepared mustard
  salt and pepper to taste

Preheat oven to 450°.

Wipe meat with damp cloth. (Lamb usually has a thick coating on the fat side. Ask your butcher to remove it or you could remove it yourself with a sharp knife.)

Cut small gashes in meat and insert minced garlic. Cover with mustard. Sprinkle with salt and pepper. Place meat fat side up in shallow roasting pan. Adjust heat to 325°. Roast meat 30 minutes per pound (20 minutes per pound if you prefer it rare).

Before serving, slice lamb and spoon pan juices over it.

Total Grams 4.7
Grams per serving 1.2

Stuffed Lamb from the Greek Isles

8 servings

2 tablespoons butter or
  margarine
1 pound ground veal or
  ground beef
3 tablespoons chopped
  onion
1 clove garlic, minced
½ cup white wine
1 8-ounce can tomato
  sauce

1 tablespoon dill
1 tablespoon chopped
  parsley
½ cup grated Parmesan
  cheese
salt and pepper to taste
1 leg of lamb or breast,
  boned and flattened

Preheat oven to 300°.

Melt 1 tablespoon butter in heavy skillet. Add ground meat, onion, and garlic, and brown lightly.

Pour wine in skillet slowly, and cook for 2 minutes. Add tomato sauce, dill, and parsley. Cook over medium heat for 10 minutes or until liquid has been absorbed. Remove from heat. Pour off fat. Sprinkle with Parmesan cheese, salt, and pepper.

Wipe lamb with damp cloth. Sprinkle with salt and pepper.

Spread ground meat mixture on lamb and roll up carefully. Use skewers to fasten it or tie with string.

Melt 1 tablespoon butter in medium-sized roasting pan. Add lamb roll. Brown over medium heat.

Place in 300° oven for 2 hours or until meat is tender. (If it seems a little dry, add 2 or 3 tablespoons water to pan.)

Total Grams 29.5
Grams per serving 3.5

Lamb and Zucchini in Sauce

4 servings

4 tablespoons butter or
   margarine
2 pounds lamb cut into
   2-inch pieces
2 tablespoons chopped
   onion
1 clove garlic (optional)
1¼ cups water plus 2
   tablespoons

salt and pepper to
   taste
1 pound zucchini, sliced
1 teaspoon cumin
1 egg
2 tablespoons lemon
   juice

In medium-sized pot melt butter or margarine. Add lamb that has been washed, and sauté until lightly browned.

Add onion and garlic. Sauté for 5 minutes.

Add ½ cup water, salt, and pepper. Simmer for about 45 minutes until water is absorbed.

Add zucchini, cumin, and ¾ cup water. Simmer until liquid is absorbed.

To make sauce, in bowl beat together egg, 2 tablespoons water, and lemon juice. Stir in drippings from lamb. Beat well. Pour sauce over lamb mixture. Do not stir.

Shake pan gently over low heat until sauce begins to thicken.

Total Grams   21.0
Grams per serving   5.2

Also good with eggplant in place of zucchini.

Moussaka

6 servings

3 tablespoons butter
1 large onion, minced
½ cup chopped
  mushrooms
1 teaspoon seasoned salt
1½ pounds ground steak
1 clove garlic, minced
1 8-ounce can tomato
  sauce

½ cup cold water
¼ teaspoon nutmeg
1 medium eggplant,
  peeled and sliced
  thin
½ cup vegetable oil
½ cup grated Parmesan
  cheese

Preheat oven to 350°.

In large skillet melt butter. Sprinkle onion and mushrooms with salt and sauté in butter. Add meat and garlic. Sauté until brown (about 10 minutes), stirring occasionally. Pour in tomato sauce and water. Add nutmeg. Allow to simmer for about 15 more minutes.

While meat is cooking, slice eggplant and put in bowl of cold water. Place plate on top of bowl and let eggplant soak for 10 to 15 minutes. Dry eggplant well.

Heat vegetable oil until very hot. Fry eggplant on both sides until transparent. Drain on paper towels.

Place about half of eggplant slices on bottom of baking dish. Spread with half the meat mixture; repeat layers. Sprinkle top with Parmesan cheese. Bake in 350° oven for 30 minutes.

Total Grams 39.9
Grams per serving 6.8

Greek for delicious.

Blue Cheese Steak

6 servings

1 teaspoon ground ginger	3 pounds steak
1 teaspoon seasoned salt	¾ cup soy sauce (without
½ teaspoon dry mustard	sugar)
⅓ cup-equivalent brown	2 cloves garlic
sugar substitute	blue cheese

Combine all ingredients except cheese in glass or pottery bowl. Marinate for 24 hours in refrigerator. Remove steak from marinade and broil.

Place bits of cheese on top of steak. Place under broiler again for a moment or serve as is.

Total Grams 9.0
Grams per serving 1.5

A really different taste!

Marinated Beef Kabobs

4 servings

4 small cube steaks (approximately 2 pounds) about ¾ inch thick
1 recipe Beef Marinade (see next page)
1 small green pepper
1 cup whole fresh mushrooms
6 cherry tomatoes (½ cup)

Cut meat into 1½-inch cubes and marinate overnight in refrigerator.

Drop pepper and mushrooms in pan of boiling water and cook for 2 minutes. Drain.

Place meat and vegetables on skewers. Broil 4 inches from heat (about 6 minutes per side for well done).

Beef Marinade
- ½ cup water
- ⅔ cup soy protein seasoning
- ¼ cup-equivalent sugar substitute
- 1 tablespoon ground ginger
- ½ teaspoon garlic powder

Total Grams	24.0
Grams per serving	6.0

Soaked with socko flavor!

Beef Stroganoff

6 servings

- 3 medium onions, chopped
- ½ pound mushrooms, sliced
- ¼ pound butter
- 1½ pounds steak, cut into finger-size strips
- ⅛ teaspoon tarragon
- 2 teaspoons dry mustard
- 1½ teaspoons seasoned salt
- ½ cup sour cream
- 1 tablespoon dry sherry
- 1 bay leaf

chives

Sauté onions and mushrooms in butter until soft and golden, and remove to casserole. Brown meat in remaining butter, but do not cook through. Place browned beef in casserole with onions and mushrooms.

To remaining juices in same pan, add tarragon, mustard, salt, 1 tablespoon sour cream, and sherry. Mix well, and pour over beef, onions, and mushrooms. Stir all ingredients until well blended. Bury bay leaf in beef, and simmer over very low heat for 25 minutes.

Remove bay leaf, add remaining sour cream, and mix well. Garnish with chives.

This should be served on top of 1 recipe Pasta (see Index), shaped into thin noodles.

Total Grams 27.3
Grams per serving 4.6

Ivan the Terrible never had it so good!

Steak Pizzaiola

6 servings

⅛ cup vegetable oil
¼ cup olive oil
2 tablespoons tarragon vinegar
1 teaspoon water freshly cracked black pepper
3 pounds sirloin steak
8 Italian plum tomatoes, cut into strips (1 cup)

2 cloves garlic, crushed
1 tablespoon chopped parsley
1 teaspoon oregano
⅛ teaspoon seasoned salt
4 tablespoons pine nuts
⅛ teaspoon-equivalent sugar substitute

Combine vegetable oil with ⅛ cup olive oil, vinegar, water, and pepper. Place steak in mixture and marinate in refrigerator for at least 2 hours, preferably overnight.

Heat remaining olive oil, and add tomatoes, garlic, parsley, oregano, salt, and pine nuts. Cook over medium heat for 3 minutes. Remove from heat, add sugar substitute, and keep warm.

Broil steak to your favorite doneness, slice, and pour mixture over it. Serve immediately.

Total Grams 17.6
Grams per serving 2.9

Something special for company!

Our Steak, Italiano

8 servings

1 oyster cut London broil
1 tablespoon vegetable oil
garlic powder
1 medium eggplant, sliced and peeled
bowl salted water
5 tablespoons olive oil
1½ sweet red peppers, cored, seeded, cut into strips, marinated in vinegar
1 green pepper, cored, seeded, cut into strips
½ cup pitted black olives
½ teaspoon seasoned salt
2 shallots, chopped (about 2 tablespoons)
2 teaspoons tomato paste
½ cup dry white wine
1 package meat broth dissolved in ¼ cup water

Rub London broil with vegetable oil and garlic powder.

Place eggplant in salted water, cover with heavy dish (to hold eggplant down), and allow to stand for ½ hour.

Rinse eggplant and drain well on paper towels.

Heat 4 tablespoons olive oil and fry eggplant on both sides until soft and transparent, removing from pan as cooked. Sauté peppers until they begin to soften (a short time).

Put eggplant back into pan with peppers. Add olives and salt. Simmer until olives are heated through. Keep warm.

Cook London broil to desired doneness. Slice.

Cook shallots in 1 tablespoon warm olive oil for 1 minute. Add tomato paste, wine, and broth, and bring to a boil. Remove from heat.

Spoon eggplant mixture over steak; add shallot mixture. Serve immediately.

Total Grams   43.7
Grams per serving   5.4

For those who like their steak with an Italian flavor!

Cabbage Rolls Stuffed with Meat (Dolma)

6 servings

1 medium cabbage	4 tablespoons chopped
1½ pounds ground lamb	parsley
or beef	2 eggs
4 tablespoons diced	1 teaspoon salt
onion	pepper to taste

⅓ cup tomato sauce

Sauce
1 cup chopped cabbage
½ cup water
⅔ can tomato sauce (8 ounces)
½ teaspoon sour salt (citric acid)
2 tablespoons lemon juice
1½ teaspoon-equivalents sugar substitute

Clean cabbage and remove any damaged leaves.

Pour boiling water over cabbage. Cover and let stand for ½ hour.

Mix ground meat, onion, parsley, eggs, salt, pepper, and tomato sauce together.

Drain cabbage, core, and separate leaves.

To Stuff: Use 12 leaves. Put 2 full tablespoons of meat mixture in center of each leaf. Bring sides up over filling and roll leaf up. Set aside.

Sauce: Chop remaining cabbage (the core and leaves not suitable for stuffing).

Place water in large Dutch oven or large kettle. Bring to boil. Add chopped cabbage, tomato sauce, sour salt, lemon juice, and sugar substitute. Turn heat down. Simmer for 15 minutes, covered.

Remove 1 cup sauce and set aside. Place cabbage rolls in pan as close together as possible. Pour cup of sauce over cabbage rolls. Cover. Simmer for 1½ hours.

Total Grams 50
Grams per serving 8.3

Extra work, but extra good!

Pot Roast from the South of Italy

6 servings

⅓ cup red wine
4 tablespoons sliced onion
5 cloves garlic
2 teaspoons basil
1 teaspoon oregano
1 tablespoon parsley

½ cup olive oil
salt and pepper
5-pound rump, chuck, or round roast
1 8-ounce can tomato sauce
sugar substitute to taste

In a bowl combine wine, onion, garlic, basil, oregano, parsley, ⅓ cup olive oil, salt, and pepper. Add meat and turn several times in mixture until meat is completely covered with marinade. Cover bowl, and keep in refrigerator for 1 day, turning meat twice. Remove meat from marinade and dry well.

Boil marinade until it reduces to about half the volume. Brown roast in remaining olive oil. Pour reduced marinade over meat. Cover and simmer for about 2 hours.

Add tomato sauce and sugar substitute. Simmer for ½ hour, or until tender when tested with fork.

Remove meat from pan. Skim off excess fat, and use remaining sauce as gravy. (This is done more easily if chilled first, as fat will harden on surface.)

Slice meat and return to sauce. Warm through and serve.

Total Grams 23.6
Grams per serving 4.0

The old family recipe never tasted better!

Spicy Spareribs

4 servings

4 pounds spareribs (or beef ribs)	¾ teaspoon salt
	¼ teaspoon dry mustard
1 tablespoon paprika	¼ teaspoon garlic powder
2 teaspoons chili powder	⅛ teaspoon pepper

Preheat oven to 450°.

Place single layer of ribs, meaty side down, in shallow roasting pan. Roast in 450° oven for ½ hour. Drain off fat.

Combine rest of ingredients. Place in saltshaker. Sprinkle evenly over ribs.

Reduce oven to 350°. Roast, meaty side up, for spareribs, ½ to 1 hour longer. (Beef ribs will take about 1 hour longer.)

Total Grams Trace
Grams per serving 0

A diet pleasure!

Oriental Spareribs

4 servings

¼ cup soy protein
seasoning
1 teaspoon ginger
1½ teaspoons sherry
extract
3 cloves garlic, minced

1 teaspoon orange
extract
3 tablespoon-
equivalents brown
sugar substitute
1 cup water

4 pounds spareribs

Preheat oven to 350°.

Mix first 7 ingredients to make marinade. Cut spare-ribs into serving pieces. Pour marinade over spareribs. Refrigerate overnight.

Place ribs and marinade in roasting pan. Bake in 350° oven. Baste every 20 minutes until brown (about 1½ hours).

Total Grams 11.4

Grams per serving 3.6

Stuffed Steak

6 servings

garlic powder
3 pounds of your favorite
cut of steak (cut with
pockets)
½ pound mushrooms
½ teaspoon thyme
3 sprigs parsley (tops
only)

5 slices ham
2 tablespoons sweet
butter
2 shallots, finely chopped
(or 1 small onion)
1 clove garlic, chopped
2 tablespoons dry white
wine

Rub garlic powder on steak and set aside.

Finely chop together mushrooms, thyme, parsley, and ham in large wooden chopping bowl.

Heat butter over low flame until melted and bubbles disappear. Brown shallots and garlic in butter. Add mushroom mixture and cook for 3 minutes, stirring occasionally. Add wine and cook 1 more minute.

Remove from heat and spoon mushroom mixture into pockets in steak. Stuff firmly, and sew closed with a trussing needle and thread.

Broil steak to desired doneness.

Serve with hot Parsley Butter Sauce (see Index)

Total Grams	18.6
Grams per serving	3.1
Grams for parsley butter per serving	.9

A pocketful of taste!

Short Ribs in Rich Beef Broth

4 servings

4 tablespoons bacon fat
3 pounds short ribs of beef
½ cup diced onion
¾ cup diced celery
3 cloves garlic

2 cups beef bouillon
salt and pepper to taste
½ recipe Frozen Horse-radish Cream (see Index)

In heavy skillet heat fat. Put ribs in skillet, and brown on all sides. Remove ribs from heat, and keep warm.

Sauté onion and celery in same fat until onion is golden. Add garlic. Cook for 2 more minutes. Place ribs back in pan and pour bouillon over them. Add salt and pepper. Simmer for 3 hours or until meat pulls away from bone easily.

Serve meat on plate with horseradish cream. Serve broth separately. (You may prefer to serve meat in broth, in which you first melt horseradish cream.)

Total Grams 24.2
Grams per serving 6.0

A good hearty meal that means economy plus in terms of money; satisfaction plus in terms of taste.

Corned Beef and Cabbage

6 servings

4 or 5 pounds corned beef
1 clove garlic
6 tablespoons sliced onion
1 small head cabbage (about 4 cups)

Wash beef and place in enough cold water to cover meat.

Bring water to boil and remove foam from surface with shallow spoon. Add garlic clove. Cover.

Reduce heat and simmer for about 3 hours or until meat is tender. Add onion and cook for 30 more minutes.

Add cabbage, which has been cut into 6 equal portions, and cook for 10 to 15 minutes or until tender.

Remove to heated platter. Slice meat and serve with cabbage.

Total Grams 47.1
Grams per serving 7.8

Delicious served with horseradish or mustard.

Cold Spiced Beef

6 servings

2 cups julienne strips
  leftover roast beef
2 medium onions, sliced
½ cup olive oil
¼ cup wine vinegar
4 tablespoons capers
2 tablespoons chopped
  parsley

2 teaspoons chopped
  chives
2 teaspoon tarragon
¼ teaspoon dry mustard
2 teaspoons basil (or
  chervil)
8 drops Tabasco sauce
salt and pepper

Combine all ingredients, mixing well.

Let stand at room temperature for 4 hours.

Stir. Chill thoroughly before serving.

Total Grams   20.9
Grams per serving   3.5

Warm your taste buds!

Meat Loaf

6 servings

3 pounds chopped meat
2 teaspoons chili powder
3 eggs
¼ teaspoon garlic powder
  olive oil

1 teaspoon onion powder
2 tablespoons parsley
1 8-ounce can tomato
  sauce

Preheat oven to 350°.

In a large bowl thoroughly mix first 6 ingredients.
Add ½ can tomato sauce and mix well.

Shape meat into loaf and place in oiled loaf pan. Bake in moderate 350° oven for 1 hour.

Pour remaining tomato sauce on top of meat loaf and bake for ½ hour more, basting occasionally.

Total Grams 19.7
Grams per serving 3.3

Also very tasty served cold.

Meat Loaf with a Middle

2 servings

1 pound chopped meat
1 teaspoon seasoned salt
¼ teaspoon poultry seasoning
1 teaspoon mustard
½ cup shredded Cheddar cheese
1 small tomato, sliced thinly

Place meat in bowl. Add salt and poultry seasoning and mix well.

Divide meat into 2 parts. Shape each into an oval and place on waxed paper. Spread mustard on each oval. Place cheese and tomato on one oval of meat. Place rest of meat on top and press edges together to seal. Broil for 15 minutes on 1 side and 10 minutes on the other until done.

Total Grams 8.0
Grams per serving 4.0

Bursting with flavor!

Mushroom Meat Loaf

4 to 6 servings

1 3-ounce can chopped
   mushrooms
1 egg, slightly beaten
1½ teaspoons Worcester-
   shire sauce
1 teaspoon salt

½ teaspoon dry mustard
   dash of pepper
½ teaspoon poultry
   seasoning
1½ pounds very lean
   ground beef

Preheat oven to 350°.

Mix all ingredients except meat. Add beef, and mix
lightly but thoroughly. Form into loaf and center in
13 x 9 x 2 pan. Bake in 350° oven for 1 to 1¼ hours.

Total Grams 4.4
Grams per serving 1.1

Meatballs in Tomato Sauce

6 servings

4 tablespoons diced onion
3 tablespoons diced green
   pepper
3 cloves garlic, diced fine
4 tablespoons olive oil
1 pound sausage meat
   (preferably Italian
   sweet or hot)

2 pounds chopped beef
2 eggs, lightly beaten
1 teaspoon thyme
1 teaspoon parsley
3 tablespoons grated
   Parmesan cheese
1 cup bouillon
1 cup tomato sauce

In saucepan sauté 3 tablespoons onion, green pepper,
and 2 cloves garlic in olive oil until light brown.
Reserve drippings in pan.

Remove sausage from casings and place in bowl with
chopped beef. Add sautéed vegetables, eggs, thyme,
parsley, and Parmesan cheese. Mix well. Roll into
2-inch balls.

Add meatballs to drippings in saucepan. Sauté until brown on all sides. (Add more oil if they stick.) Remove from pan.

Sauté 1 tablespoon onion and 1 clove garlic in saucepan until light brown.

Add bouillon and tomato sauce. Simmer for 12 minutes.

Place meatballs back in pan, stirring carefully. Do not break up meatballs. Simmer for 5 more minutes.

> Total Grams   28.0
> Grams per serving   4.5

Double the recipe and freeze half of it for handy use another time!

Fromage Burgers

6 servings

2 pounds ground lean beef
1 tablespoon chopped chives
¾ teaspoon crumbled tarragon
2 teaspoons seasoned salt
¼ cup chopped fresh parsley

¼ cup chopped scallions
1 egg, beaten
6 slices American, Swiss, or blue cheese
3 tablespoons butter, melted

Combine beef, chives, tarragon, salt, parsley, scallions, and egg.

Shape into 12 equal balls. Flatten each ball to pancake shape.

Place cheese on 6 of the meat pancakes. Place other meat on top and press edges together to seal.

Brush each with melted butter and broil to desired doneness, turning once.

Total Grams 13.8
Grams per serving 2.3

Two-for-one!

Pizza Burgers

6 servings

2 pounds ground beef
1 teaspoon seasoned salt
1 tablespoon chopped
   parsley
⅛ teaspoon basil
⅛ teaspoon oregano
2 eggs, beaten
1 package fried pork
   rinds, crushed

¼ cup salad oil
6 slices mozzarella cheese
½ recipe Pasta Sauce
   (see Index)
2 tablespoons grated
   Parmesan cheese

Preheat oven to 400°.

Toss chopped meat with salt, parsley, basil, and oregano.

Shape into 6 patties ½ inch thick.

Dip patties into eggs and then into pork rinds. Sauté patties in hot oil until well browned on both sides. Arrange in shallow baking dish. Top each patty with a piece of mozzarella cheese. Pour on pasta sauce. Sprinkle with Parmesan cheese.

Bake in 400° oven for 25 minutes.

Total Grams 46.2
Grams per serving 7.7

Kids will love them.

Chili

6 servings

4 tablespoons olive oil
½ cup sliced onion
2 cloves garlic, minced
3 pounds hamburger

2 8-ounce cans tomato
   sauce
2 teaspoons chili powder
1 teaspoon cumin

1½ teaspoons salt

Heat oil in skillet. Sauté onion for about 3 minutes. Add garlic and sauté until light brown. Push onion and garlic to side of pan.

Add hamburger in one piece, and as it browns break it up slowly. (This is done to allow meat to retain its juices.)

When hamburger is slightly browned, add tomato sauce, chili powder, cumin, and salt. Simmer for 15 minutes.

Total Grams   41.3
Grams per serving   7.0

Sausage and Peppers

8 servings

3 pounds Italian sweet sausage
2 pounds green peppers
5 tablespoons olive oil
½ cup sliced onion
4 cloves garlic, minced

Sauté sausages in skillet until well browned on all sides. Wash green peppers, remove seeds, and cut into quarters.

Heat olive oil in heavy frypan. Add peppers and onion. Cook over low heat for 10 minutes. Stir often. Add garlic. Cook for 4 more minutes.

Remove sausages from skillet. Drain well. Cut into 1-inch slices. Add to green peppers and onion. Stir well. Cook for 10 more minutes.

Total Grams 48.6
Grams per serving 6.1

Sausage and Peppers with Tomato Sauce: Add 1 8-ounce can tomato sauce to above recipe. Simmer gently.

Total Grams 61.4
Grams per serving 7.7

Very, very good—but watch your carbohydrates!

Sausage-Pepper Stuff

6 servings

3 large green peppers
1½ pounds Italian sweet sausage (removed from casings)
2 tablespoons butter
½ large onion, chopped
½ eggplant, peeled and cubed

½ cup heavy cream
⅛ teaspoon thyme
⅛ teaspoon oregano
⅛ teaspoon rosemary
⅛ teaspoon marjoram
⅛ teaspoon basil
pinch of ground sage

Halve each pepper. Remove core and seeds. Place in large pot of boiling salted water. Parboil for 8 minutes. Drain and keep warm.

Place sausage in large skillet. Brown well. Remove from pan and pour off grease.

Melt butter in skillet. Add onion and eggplant. Sauté until onion is golden. Add cooked sausage. Cool.

Add heavy cream to skillet with spices. Mix well. Heat slowly. Stir well. Do not allow to boil.

Spoon sausage mixture into pepper halves. Serve hot.

Total Grams 23.5
Grams per serving 4.0

More taste than carbohydrates!

Pizza with Meat Crust

6 servings

1 pound ground beef
⅛ cup grated Parmesan
cheese
¼ cup beef bouillon
1 onion, chopped
1 clove garlic, minced
1 teaspoon seasoned salt

1 8-ounce can tomato
sauce
1 cup ricotta cheese,
drained
2 egg yolks, beaten
½ cup mozzarella cheese
in thin slices

16 slices pepperoni

Preheat oven to 375°.

Mix beef, Parmesan cheese, bouillon, onion, garlic, and salt together well. Press into 9-inch pie plate to form shell.

Bake in 375° oven for 15 minutes. Remove from oven and pour off excess fat.

Combine tomato sauce, ricotta, and egg yolks. Fill meat shell.

Top with mozzarella slices and pepperoni.

Lower oven heat to 325°. Bake for 40 minutes.

Total Grams 37.3
Grams per serving 6.2

You can eat it—crust and all!

POULTRY

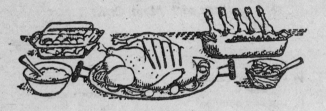

Chicken in Sauce

4 servings

3 pounds chicken for
 frying, cut into
 pieces
salt
4 tablespoons oil
½ pound mushrooms

2 tablespoons onion,
 minced
2 tablespoons tomato
 sauce
2 teaspoons lemon juice
½ cup white wine

Sprinkle chicken pieces with salt.

Heat oil in skillet, add pieces of chicken, and sauté
well on all sides. Remove to dish and keep warm.

Sauté mushrooms and onion until onion is soft. Add
tomato sauce, lemon juice, and wine, bring to a boil,
stirring constantly.

Pour sauce over chicken.

Total Grams 20.8
Grams per serving 5.2

Leftover Curry

6 servings

1 large onion, diced
2 tablespoons oil
4½ cups cubed chicken
 or ham, cooked
½ cup boiling water

1 package chicken
 bouillon
½ teaspoon curry
 powder
lettuce

In large skillet sauté onion in oil until golden. Add
chicken or ham. Combine water and bouillon. Pour in

skillet. Add curry powder and simmer for 10 minutes.
Serve on bed of lettuce.

Total Grams 16.4
Grams per serving 2.7

You would never know they were leftovers!

Chicken Cacciatora

8 servings

5 pounds spring chicken,
cut into pieces or
breasts, legs, and
thighs equaling 5
pounds
½ cup olive oil
4 tablespoons butter
⅓ cup chopped onion
1 2½-ounce jar mush-
rooms

3 cloves garlic
¾ cup dry white wine
2 bay leaves
1 teaspoon basil
½ teaspoon freshly
ground black
pepper
5 tablespoons tomato
sauce
salt to taste

2 tablespoons brandy

Sauté chicken in olive oil until light brown.

Heat butter in skillet. When it stops bubbling, add
onion and sauté until golden. Add mushrooms, reserving liquid they are packed in. Add garlic. Cook
for 4 more minutes. Spoon mushrooms and onions
over chicken. Pour in wine. Add bay leaves, basil, and
pepper. Simmer for about 8 minutes, uncovered.

Stir in tomato sauce and mushroom liquid. Salt to
taste. Cook, uncovered, for 20 more minutes.

Add brandy, and serve.

Total Grams 24.5
Grams per serving 3.0

Surprisingly quick and easy!

Cheddar and Chicken

6 servings

½ pound mushrooms, chopped
8 tablespoons butter
½ cup heavy cream
2 cups shredded Cheddar cheese
1 teaspoon seasoned salt
½ teaspoon cayenne pepper

6 chicken breasts, split, boned, and skinless
4 eggs, beaten
1 2¾-ounce bag chopped pork rinds, chopped fine
½ cup dry white wine

Preheat oven to 325°.

Sauté mushrooms in 4 tablespoons butter until well browned. Add heavy cream, cheese, salt, and pepper. Stir until cheese melts. Remove from heat and place in freezer until mixture becomes solid. Remove from freezer and slice into 12 equal pieces.

Place 1 piece of cheese in center of each chicken breast. Roll breasts and tie with string. Dip in eggs and then in pork rinds.

In skillet brown chicken rolls in 4 tablespoons melted butter. Transfer chicken rolls and butter to baking dish, and pour wine in dish. Bake in 350° oven for 45 minutes, basting occasionally.

Total Grams 21.7
Grams per serving 3.6

A really special main dish for really special occasions!

Absolutely Fabulous Roast Chicken

4 servings

  seasoned salt
  garlic powder
1 roasting chicken
¼ pound sweet butter, at room temperature

Preheat oven to 450°.

Sprinkle salt and garlic powder on chicken inside and out. Allow to sit for at least 1 hour.

Rub butter on chicken, making a thick coating. Sprinkle on more salt. Place in baking pan that has been lined with large strips of foil.

Wrap foil around chicken so no steam can escape. Bake in 450° oven for 1 hour. Turn down to 325° and bake until tender, for at least 1 more hour.

Total Grams   .8
Grams per serving   .2

The name says it all!

Teriyaki Broiled Chicken

6 servings

12 chicken legs and thighs or 6 broiler halves
½ cup olive oil
⅓ cup soy protein seasoning
1 tablespoon-equivalent
brown sugar substitute
1 tablespoon grated orange rind
1 tablespoon ginger
2 cloves garlic
⅓ cup sherry
oil for brushing

Place chicken in shallow baking dish. Make marinade by blending rest of ingredients. Pour marinade over chicken.

Refrigerate for about 6 hours or overnight. Turn occasionally.

Place chicken in broiler about 5 to 6 inches from heat (any closer and it will burn). Brush with small amount of oil.

Spoon marinade over chicken several times during broiling. Broil to desired doneness.

Total Grams   7.2
Grams per serving 1.2

For those who like their chicken Japanese style!

Cannelloni with Chicken

4 servings (8 crepes)

3 chicken livers
1 boned chicken breast
4 tablespoons butter
5 slices prosciutto
¼ teaspoon marjoram
¾ cup grated Parmesan
   cheese

1 recipe Cream Sauce
   (see Index)
8 crepes (Pasta recipe,
   see Index)

Preheat oven to 350°.

Sauté chicken livers and chicken breast in 2 table-spoons butter until brown on both sides.

Grind livers, chicken, and prosciutto in food grinder with medium blade. Mix in marjoram and ½ cup grated Parmesan cheese. Add 10 tablespoons cream sauce. Place 2 tablespoons chicken mixture in center of each crepe. Roll crepes up.

Butter baking dish with 2 tablespoons softened butter. Place crepes in buttered dish. Cover with remaining cream sauce and Parmesan cheese.

Bake in 350° oven for ½ hour.

Total Grams 29.8
Grams per serving 3.7

Complicated but worth the effort!

Lemon Basted Roast Chicken

4 servings

1 chicken, cut up
½ teaspoon oregano
¼ teaspoon garlic powder
¼ cup butter (½ stick)
salt and pepper
juice of 2 lemons (6 to 8 tablespoons)

Preheat oven to 400°.

Sprinkle chicken with oregano and garlic powder. Melt butter in roasting pan or casserole. Roll chicken in it. Sprinkle with salt and pepper.

Roast chicken skin side up, uncovered, in 400° oven for 30 minutes or until golden brown. Turn pieces over and continue roasting until brown (about 30 more minutes).

Reduce heat to 300° and cook until tender. Squeeze lemon juice over chicken.

Cover and let sit in turned-off oven for 15 minutes. Remove to platter and serve.

Total Grams 9.3
Grams per serving 2.3

A delicious dinner with a salad and green vegetable!

Coq au Vin

8 servings

4 slices thick-sliced bacon	dissolved in 1 cup water
7 tablespoons butter	¼ teaspoon garlic powder
4 pounds chicken, cut up	¼ teaspoon thyme
1 teaspoon seasoned salt	1 bay leaf
¼ cup cognac (or brandy)	4 medium-sized onions, sliced
1 cup dry red wine	1 pound mushrooms
2 packages dry broth	chopped chives

Dice bacon and sauté in 4 tablespoons butter until brown. Remove from skillet and save.

Wash and thoroughly dry chicken. Brown in bacon fat and season. Put bacon back in pan, cover, and simmer for about 10 minutes.

Heat cognac in small pan. Ignite, and pour over chicken. Add wine, broth, garlic powder, and thyme. Bury bay leaf in chicken, cover, and simmer for 45 minutes. Remove chicken and keep warm. Boil liquid in pan until it reduces by half.

Sauté onions and mushrooms in 3 tablespoons butter until onions are golden.

Put chicken back into skillet with mushrooms and onions around it. Simmer for 5 minutes. Garnish with chives and serve.

Total Grams 58.5
Grams per serving 7.4

A gourmet's taste delight!

Chicken à la Firenze

4 servings

4 boneless chicken breasts	1 clove garlic, crushed
2 eggs, beaten	dash of marjoram
½ package fried pork rinds, crushed	dash of basil
3 tablespoons butter	⅓ cup cream
½ cup Sauterne	½ pound spinach, cooked *
1 cup chicken broth or bouillon	¼ cup grated Parmesan cheese

Preheat oven to 350°.

Dip chicken in eggs and then into pork rinds until well coated. Sauté in butter until chicken begins to brown. Turn once. Lower heat. Add wine and cook until wine has almost evaporated. Remove from heat.

Mix together broth, garlic, marjoram, basil, and cream to make a sauce.

Place ½ spinach in bottom of casserole. Add chicken and rest of spinach. Pour sauce over top. Sprinkle with Parmesan cheese and bake in 350° oven for ½ hour.

Total Grams 18.5
Grams per serving 4.6

* To cook fresh spinach: Wash carefully several times to remove all sand. Place in pot with just enough water to cover it. Cook at low boil for about 20 minutes or until tender, but not limp. Press out water before serving.

Two packages of frozen spinach may be substituted for fresh spinach. Cook to package directions. Whether fresh or frozen, do not overcook.

Chicken and Almonds

8 servings

½ pound mushrooms, sliced
1 green pepper, chopped
½ cup butter
½ teaspoon seasoned salt
4 cups diced chicken
½ cup dry white wine
2 cups heavy cream
2 egg yolks, beaten
nutmeg
6 thin slices Swiss cheese
¼ cup sliced almonds

Sauté mushrooms and pepper in butter until soft. Sprinkle with salt and add chicken.

Stir in wine and cook until liquid reduces to about half. Add heavy cream and scald mixture. (Bring it just to boiling point, but do not boil.) Beat in egg yolks and continue to cook, stirring constantly, for about 5 minutes until liquid begins to thicken. Season to taste with more salt and nutmeg.

Place in casserole. Cover chicken with cheese and sprinkle almonds on top. Place under broiler. Broil until cheese melts.

Total Grams 43.5
Grams per serving 5.5

Twice as good the day after!

Summer Day Chicken from Spain

4 servings

1 3-pound chicken, or
 favorite chicken
 pieces
¼ cup corn or safflower
 oil
2 cloves garlic
 juice of 1 lemon
1 teaspoon grated
 orange rind

2 bay leaves
½ cup vinegar
1 cup white wine
1 cup chicken broth
½ teaspoon coarsely
 ground pepper
salt to taste

Clean chicken. Heat oil in skillet. Lightly brown chicken on medium heat.

Combine remaining ingredients for marinade. Pour over chicken.

Simmer, covered, for 1 hour. Add more broth, if necessary, to keep chicken covered.

When chicken is done, place in refrigerator, covered with marinade. Serve cold in sauce.

Total Grams 23.3
Grams per serving 6.0

Austrian Paprika Chicken

6 servings

2 tablespoons butter
2 tablespoons vegetable
 oil
2 chickens (broilers), cut
 up
 seasoned salt

4 small onions
1 clove garlic, minced
2 tablespoons paprika
 (from a freshly
 opened jar)
1 cup chicken broth

1 cup sour cream

Preheat oven to 350°.

Heat butter and oil together. Brown chicken carefully in oil on all sides. Add salt. Remove chicken from pan.

Place onions and garlic in fat and sauté until onions are golden. Add paprika, broth, and sour cream. Stir constantly until mixture is smooth.

Place chicken in casserole and cover with mixture, making sure to scrape pan well of all drippings.

Bake, covered, in 350° oven for 1 hour.

Serve with Tossed Salad with Tomato Dressing (see Index).

Total Grams   21.7
Grams per serving   4.6

At home in any flavor setting!

Chicken Croquettes Elegante

2 servings

1½ cups ground chicken meat
2 egg whites
¼ teaspoon poultry seasoning
pinch of salt
fat for deep frying
2 tablespoons chopped onion

4 large mushrooms, chopped
1 tablespoon oil or butter
Quick Cream Sauce (see Index)

Preheat oven to 375°.

Mix chicken, egg whites, poultry seasoning, and salt. Form into croquettes 1 inch wide and 3 inches long. Fry in deep fat until crisp.

Sauté mushrooms and onion in oil until lightly browned.

Prepare sauce.

In casserole or shirring dish place mushrooms and onions, and arrange croquettes on top.

Pour sauce on top.

Bake in 375° oven for about 8 to 10 minutes until thoroughly heated.

To make a prettier dish, place sliced hard-cooked eggs between croquettes. Then add sauce. Sprinkle with paprika.

Total Grams 5.3
Grams per serving 3.0

Gourmet Game Hens

6 servings

¾ cup butter
¾ cup white port wine
3 tablespoons dried tarragon
6 garlic cloves, peeled
1½ teaspoons salt

¾ teaspoon pepper
6 frozen Rock Cornish hens, about 1¼ pounds each, thawed
garlic powder

Preheat oven to 400°.

In saucepan melt butter. Add wine and 1 tablespoon dried tarragon.

Place 1 garlic clove, 1 teaspoon tarragon, ¼ teaspoon salt, and ⅛ teaspoon pepper in each hen. Sprinkle outside liberally with garlic powder.

Pour wine sauce over hens and roast in large shallow pan, without rack, for about 1 hour or until well browned and drumstick twists easily. Baste frequently with sauce.

Total Grams 9.2
Grams per serving 1.4

This is wonderful!

Turkey à la King

4 servings

4 egg yolks	1 cup strong chicken
¼ teaspoon seasoned salt	broth
½ teaspoon dry tarragon	2 cups diced turkey
1 cup heavy cream	meat *
nutmeg	

Preheat oven to 350°.

Beat yolks until thick and lemon-colored. Add salt and tarragon. Beat in heavy cream. Stir in broth, then add turkey meat.

Pour into 4 small oven-proof bowls. Sprinkle with nutmeg.

Set bowls in shallow pan half full with water, and bake in 350° oven for 30 minutes.

Total Grams 9.8
Grams per serving 2.7

* *For the economy minded*: Turkey drumsticks (frozen) 2 to a package may also be used. Follow cooking instructions on package.

The How-Tos of Roast Turkey

This is an easy, delicious way to cook turkey. It will never be dry.

Preheat oven to 400°.

Have turkey at room temperature. Remove giblets from cavity. Run turkey under cold water to clean inside and out. Never soak a turkey in water. Dry it well.

Rub turkey with salt inside and out. Use about ⅓ teaspoon salt per pound. Insert poultry pins to draw body opening together. Use string to lace between pins (as you would lace a shoe).

Tie legs together with string if they are not already tucked under a piece of skin. Bend wing tips under body and tuck loose neck skin under turkey.

Put 2 large pieces of aluminum foil crisscrossed in large roasting pan. Place turkey breast side up on foil. Cover turkey breast with slices of uncooked bacon.

Bring up lengths of aluminum foil and seal around turkey. It should be completely covered.

Cook in 400° oven for 20 minutes. Reduce to 350°. Cook for 15 minutes per pound if turkey is over 10 pounds. If under 10 pounds, cook for 20 minutes per pound.

Total Grams   0

Dressing: 1 recipe Almond Stuffing (see next page)

After salting inside of bird, fill body cavity loosely with stuffing.

Add 5 minutes more per pound.

Almond Stuffing

½ cup butter
½ cup finely chopped onion
¼ pound smoked ham, finely ground
¼ cup chopped parsley
½ teaspoon thyme

½ teaspoon freshly ground pepper
½ cup fried pork rinds, crushed
2 eggs
¼ cup dry red wine
⅔ cup blanched almonds

Melt butter in large skillet. Add onions. Cook until light brown. Add ham, parsley, and spices. Mix well.

Combine mixture with pork rinds, eggs, wine, and almonds.

Total Grams 41.6

Use to stuff chicken, turkey, veal roast, or anything that needs a stuffing.

FISH AND SHELLFISH

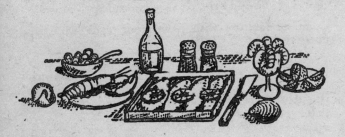

Fish in Wine Sauce

4 servings

½ stick sweet butter or margarine
½ clove garlic, chopped fine
½ cup finely chopped onion
½ teaspoon seasoned salt
4 fish fillets
1 egg, beaten
¼ cup grated Parmesan cheese
2 tablespoons dry sherry
¼ cup Sauterne

Melt butter in electric frypan. Add garlic, onion, and salt. Sauté until onion is golden brown. Set aside.

Wash and dry fish. Dip fish first into egg and then into Parmesan cheese. Place in frypan with garlic mixture and brown well on both sides. Pour wine in, cover, and simmer for 10 minutes.

Total Grams 13.0
Grams per serving 6.0

Trout in Tomato Sauce

4 servings

2 good-sized trout
5 tablespoons tomato sauce
8 tablespoons cider vinegar
3 tablespoons corn or safflower oil
1 tablespoon minced onion
4 drops Tabasco sauce (optional)
1 pinch sugar substitute

Clean and fillet trout, and cut into ½-inch pieces. Arrange attractively on shallow serving dish.

Combine remaining ingredients. Mix well. Pour over fish and cover. Place in refrigerator for 24 hours.

(If you prefer herring and it is available, use same recipe. After filleting herring, place in shallow bowl, and add cold tea enough to cover. Refrigerate overnight to remove excess salt. Follow remaining recipe.)

Total Grams 9.7
Grams per serving 2.4

Fresh Spring Salmon Mousse

10 servings

2 envelopes unflavored gelatin	½ teaspoon onion powder
1½ cups cold water	1 tablespoon capers
⅔ cup sour cream	2 teaspoons dill
1 cup mayonnaise	1 cup finely chopped peeled cucumber
1½ pounds fresh salmon, cooked, skinned, and boned	1 teaspoon salt

Soften gelatin in cold water. Heat until completely dissolved. Cool.

Mix sour cream and mayonnaise together. Add gelatin, and chill until slightly thickened.

Flake salmon and add onion powder, capers, dill, cucumber, and salt. Mix well with sour cream and mayonnaise.

Pour into 5-cup mold. Refrigerate until firm. Unmold.

Total Grams 19.6
Grams per serving 2.0

May be served with Mustard Sauce (see Index).

Broiled Fresh Salmon

2 servings

2 medium-sized fresh
salmon steaks, 1 inch
thick
lime juice
butter

salt
freshly ground black
pepper
4 pinches dried tarragon
4 ounces dry white wine

Place salmon steaks in shallow, fireproof baking pan and squeeze lime juice over them. Dot steaks liberally with butter, sprinkle with salt and pepper and a pinch (for each steak) of dried tarragon leaves. Pour wine in pan (around steaks—*not* over them).

Place pan under broiler about 4 inches from flame. Cook for about 10 to 12 minutes, basting carefully during latter part of cooking so herbs are not disturbed. Turn steaks and season as before. Broil for 5 to 6 minutes. Baste after herbs have been "set" by heat. Skin should get crisp. Watch carefully!

Total Grams   4.0
Grams per serving   2.0

Cook with care!

Savory Salmon

6 servings

½ pound mushrooms,
sliced
1 cup Sauterne
¼ cup lemon juice
2 tablespoons grated
onion
½ teaspoon seasoned salt

8 tablespoons corn oil
margarine, at room
temperature
½ teaspoon dried
tarragon
½ teaspoon minced
chives

6 salmon steaks

Marinate mushrooms in wine and lemon juice.

Cream onion, salt, margarine, tarragon, and chives together.

Melt half of onion mixture in frypan and brown salmon steaks on both sides.

When steaks are well browned, add remaining onion mixture. Add mushrooms and mushroom marinade. Cover and simmer for 15 minutes, basting often.

Total Grams 28.9
Grams per serving 4.8

Fabulous Flounder

6 servings

3 pounds flounder fillets
lemon juice
salt and pepper
1 teaspoon dried tarragon

2 cups sour cream
1 tablespoon minced chives
parsley

Preheat oven to 350°.

Spray with imitation grease baking dish just large enough to hold fish fillets. Rub fillets with lemon juice, salt, and pepper, and place in dish. Sprinkle with tarragon. Cover with sour cream and bake in 350° oven for 15 minutes.

Remove from oven, and sprinkle with chives and parsley. Serve immediately.

Total Grams 21.4
Grams per serving 3.6

The name says it all!

Fennel Sole

4 servings

4 fillets of sole
½ stick corn oil margarine, at room temperature
¼ teaspoon fennel seed
½ teaspoon lemon juice
¼ teaspoon dried tarragon

¼ clove garlic, minced
seasoned salt to taste
¼ cup safflower oil
1 teaspoon grated lemon rind
½ bay leaf

Wash and dry fish.

Combine margarine, fennel seed, lemon juice, tarragon, garlic, and salt.

Spread margarine mixture on fish fillets and roll fillets. Fasten with toothpicks.

Combine oil, lemon rind, and bay leaf in baking dish. Add fish and marinate in refrigerator for 1 hour. Turn once.

Drain fish and reserve marinade. Broil fish for 5 minutes on each side, basting frequently with marinade.

Total Grams   3.0
Grams per serving   .8

Stuffed Fish

6 servings

2 pounds fillet of flounder or sole
salt
3 slices bacon, diced
¼ pound mushrooms, sliced
¼ cup diced celery
2 tablespoons diced onion

1 clove garlic, diced fine
1 tablespoon parsley
3 tablespoons margarine, melted
½ cup white wine
¼ cup grated Parmesan cheese
paprika

Preheat oven to 350°.

Sprinkle fillets with salt. Allow to stand for about 10 minutes.

In skillet sauté bacon, mushrooms, celery, and onion until vegetables are soft and bacon is crisp. Add garlic 2 minutes before removing from heat. Remove from heat. Add parsley, and blend well.

Spread this mixture over fillets, roll up, and fasten with toothpicks.

Place 1 tablespoon melted margarine in bottom of baking dish. Place fish in it.

Pour remaining margarine over fish, and add wine.

Sprinkle with Parmesan cheese and paprika.

Bake in 350° oven for ½ hour.

Total Grams 21.4
Grams per serving 3.6

Halibut with Curry Sauce

4 servings

4 large slices halibut
 boiling water
2 teaspoons lemon juice
1 recipe Curry Sauce (see Index)
 sprinkle of paprika

Place halibut in pan. Cover with boiling water. Add lemon juice. Simmer for about 10 or 15 minutes, or until tender.

Make curry sauce.

Remove halibut with large spatula. Pour off water. Return halibut to pan. Pour curry sauce over fish, and sprinkle with paprika. Heat for 3 or 4 minutes.

To serve: Place fish on serving dish. Garnish with a little paprika.

Total Grams   13.3
Grams per serving   4.4

The curry flavor makes the difference!

Fish Oriental

2 servings

2 tablespoons butter or margarine	½ cup bean sprouts
2 tablespoons chopped onion	¼ head cabbage, shredded
3 slices boiled ham	4 fillets of flounder
1 clove garlic, minced	⅔ cup chicken broth
	dash of paprika

Preheat oven to 350°.

Melt butter in saucepan, add onion, and sauté until soft.

Add ham and garlic, and sauté for 3 minutes. Add bean sprouts, and sauté for about 3 or 4 minutes until lightly browned. Place fillets in small casserole. Add uncooked cabbage to bean sprout mixture. Spread over fillets.

Pour broth over fillets. Sprinkle with paprika. Cover dish with lid or aluminum foil and bake in 350° oven for 30 minutes.

Total Grams   13.8
Grams per serving   7.0

Fish Delish

4 servings

1½ pounds fillet of sole
  salt and pepper
2 tablespoons butter
1 tablespoon vegetable
  oil

¼ cup chopped parsley
1 clove garlic, minced
3 tablespoons lemon
  juice
¼ cup slivered almonds

Cut sole into 4 pieces. Sprinkle with salt and pepper.

Combine butter and oil in skillet. Sauté fish in oil for about 5 minutes, turning once.

Remove from heat, and sprinkle fish with parsley, garlic, and lemon juice. Return to heat, and simmer for about 5 more minutes, or until fish flakes. Garnish with almonds.

Total Grams   14.2
Grams per serving   3.6

Unbelievably easy!

Baked Fish Loaf

6 servings

2 cups canned tuna fish
  or salmon or 1
  pound filleted fish,
  cooked
2 teaspoons diced
  onion
2 teaspoons capers

1 cup mayonnaise
½ cup water
½ cup cream
½ teaspoon salt
¼ teaspoon paprika
½ teaspoon curry (more
  if desired)

Preheat oven to 350°.

Drain and flake fish. Add onion and capers to fish.

In a saucepan combine mayonnaise, water, cream, salt, paprika, and stir until smooth.

Add half of cream sauce to fish and mix. Place fish mixture in buttered loaf pan or baking dish. Bake in 350° oven for 30 minutes.

Add curry to remaining sauce. To serve, slice fish loaf and spoon sauce over it.

Total Grams 9.9
Grams per serving 1.6

It's the sauce that counts!

Crabmeat Almond Pie

8 servings

¼ cup chopped Toasted Almonds (see Index)
2 eggs plus 2 yolks
2 teaspoons Dijon mustard
2 teaspoons seasoned salt

2 tablespoons minced chives
2 cups grated Fontina cheese
4 ounces frozen or canned crabmeat
1½ cups heavy cream

Preheat oven to 300°.

Place toasted almonds on bottom of 9-inch pie plate.

Put eggs in bowl and beat well. Add mustard, salt, chives, cheese, and crabmeat.

Scald heavy cream by bringing it just to boiling point (do not boil). Add heavy cream to crabmeat mixture and pour into pie plate.

Bake in 300° oven for 1 hour.

Total Grams 40.7
Grams per serving 5.1

A little expensive—but impressive!

Shrimp Scampi

6 servings

1 teaspoon salt	2 pounds fresh shrimp, shelled
1 bay leaf	8 tablespoons butter
5 allspice berries	6 cloves garlic, minced
¼ teaspoon dried tarragon	4 shallots or scallions, minced
1 teaspoon white vinegar	

Heat large pot of water. Add salt, bay leaf, allspice, tarragon, and vinegar. Bring to boil. Add shrimp. Boil for 8 minutes. Drain.

Melt butter in skillet, and add garlic and shallots. Brown for 3 minutes. Add shrimp. Cook for 5 more minutes. Turn once. Serve.

Total Grams 19.6
Grams per serving 3.3

An all-time favorite—all-time good!

Shrimp in Wine

6 servings

1½ pounds fresh shrimp
1 cup dry white wine
¼ cup butter
¼ cup dry sherry

½ teaspoon garlic powder
¼ cup grated Parmesan cheese

salt to taste

Marinate shrimp in white wine for 2 hours. Remove from marinade.

Melt butter in large skillet. Add shrimp, and pour in sherry. Sprinkle with garlic powder. Allow to simmer for 10 minutes.

Add Parmesan cheese and salt. Serve warm.

Total Grams 11.7
Grams per serving 2.0

Low carbohydrates!

Shrimp Curry with Eggs

6 servings

5 tablespoons butter
1 pound boiled shrimp
or 16-ounce can
shrimp
1 cup mayonnaise

⅔ cup water
½ cup cream
1 teaspoon curry powder (more if desired)
½ teaspoon cayenne

6 eggs

In skillet melt 2 tablespoons butter. Add shrimp. Stir over moderate heat for 3 minutes. Remove from heat.

In saucepan heat mayonnaise, ½ cup water, cream, curry powder, and cayenne. Stir until smooth. Taste test—add more curry powder if desired.

Add shrimp to curry sauce, stirring lightly.

For Scrambled Eggs: Break eggs into bowl, add remaining water, and stir well.

Heat 3 tablespoons butter in skillet over moderate heat. Add eggs and stir. Allow to set, stirring again. Repeat until eggs are done.

Place about 2 tablespoons scrambled eggs in serving dish for each portion, and about 2 tablespoons of shrimp and curry sauce over eggs.

Total Grams 18.3
Grams per serving 3.0

Scrambled eggs instead of rice—delicious!

Broiled Lobster Tails with Tarragon

2 servings

4 frozen lobster tails
½ stick butter
1 tablespoon chopped or dried chives
1 teaspoon dried tarragon
½ teaspoon dry mustard
seasoned salt

Remove soft part of lobster tail with scissors. Hit hard shell slightly with mallet or cleaver to make it lie flat. Melt butter. Add chives, tarragon, mustard, and salt. Spoon generously over tails and let stand in marinade for several hours. Remove from marinade.

Broil about 4 inches from heat for 10 to 15 minutes with meaty side up. Baste often.

Total Grams 2.1
Grams per serving 1.1

Something special!

PASTAS OR SIDE DISHES

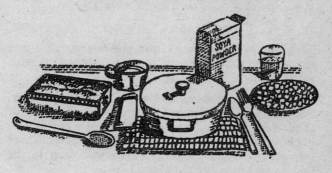

Gnocchi

8 servings

1 pound creamed
    cottage cheese or
    ricotta cheese
½ pound cream cheese
    or Boursin chcese
4 eggs, beaten
2 tablespoons soya
    powder

dash of salt, cayenne
    pepper, and nut-
    meg
½ pound sweet butter,
    melted
½ cup grated Parmesan
    cheese

Push cottage cheese and cream cheese through a fine strainer. (We find the easiest and fastest way is with your hands!)

Beat eggs into mixture with electric or rotary beater. Blend in soya powder and seasonings. Refrigerate for about 1 hour. Bring large surface pot of water to rolling boil. Lower heat to a simmer. Drop cheese mixture into water by teaspoonfuls. (They will drop to the bottom and then rise to the top.)

Allow gnocchi to poach (simmer on top of water) for about 20 minutes. Remove gnocchi carefully with slotted spoon and allow to drain on absorbent paper.

Melt ¼ pound butter in large baking dish. Place drained gnocchi in dish. Cover with remaining melted butter and grated Parmesan cheese.

Gnocchi may be served immediately, kept warm in a low oven, or refrigerated and reheated.

Total Grams   32.0
Grams per serving   4.0

The substitution of Boursin for cream cheese will give you a much spicier gnocchi. Ricotta substituted for cottage cheese gives gnocchi more body.

A perfectly delicious side dish.

Pasta

12 crepes

⅓ cup soya powder
½ cup water
3 eggs
1 tablespoon oil

Put all ingredients in blender. Blend until smooth.

Use a crepe pan or a 5- or 6-inch skillet. Cover bottom of pan lightly with small amount of oil. When pan is hot enough to sizzle a drop of water, pour about 3 tablespoons of crepe mixture into pan. Tilt pan to distribute mixture evenly. Crepes should be thin. Lightly brown on both sides (about 1 minute on each side). Place on wax paper until all crepes are finished.

These crepes are very delicate, so handle carefully. If you have trouble the first time, try again. Oil the pan again if necessary.

They could be made a day ahead and stored in the refrigerator with wax paper separating crepes.

Total Grams 24.6
Grams per crepe 2.1

A side dish standby for carbohydrate-watchers!

Mock Macaroni and Cheese

8 servings

1 pound coarsely
chopped ham
1 cup sliced mushrooms
½ cup diced onion
3 tablespoons butter
¼ teaspoon seasoned
salt

1½ cups heavy cream
2½ cups sharp grated
Cheddar cheese
½ Pasta recipe (see
Index), chopped
fine
butter

Preheat oven to 350°.

Brown ham, mushrooms, and onion in butter. Add salt. Remove from heat. Stir in heavy cream and 2 cups grated Cheddar cheese. Put back on low flame and simmer until cheese melts (do not allow to boil).

Chop pasta into small pieces and add to mixture. Mix well. Pour into buttered casserole dish. Top with remaining 1/2 cup Cheddar cheese. Bake in 350° oven for 30 minutes.

Total Grams 53.2
Grams per serving 6.7

Verrrrry special!

Manicotti

12 crepes

1/2 recipe Pasta Sauce (see Index)
1 recipe Pasta (see Index)

Stuffing for Pasta
1 pound ricotta cheese
6 ounces mozzarella cheese
2 teaspoons parsley
5 tablespoons grated Parmesan cheese
2 eggs

Preheat oven to 300°.

Prepare 7 cups pasta sauce and 12 pasta crepes.

In bowl mix ricotta cheese, mozzarella cheese, parsley, 2 tablespoons grated Parmesan cheese, and eggs.

Cover bottom of large baking pan with thin layer of pasta sauce.

Place about 2 full tablespoons of ricotta mixture in center of crepe. Roll crepe around stuffing like large noodle. Place crepe in baking pan, seam side down. Repeat with each crepe, placing them side by side in baking pan. Pour remaining sauce over top of crepes.

Sprinkle remaining 3 tablespoons Parmesan cheese on top. Bake in 300° oven for 20 minutes.

Total Grams 64.8
Grams per manicotti 7.2

This is one dish we always serve to guests—even non-dieters love this one!

Enchiladas

6 servings

Prepare 1 recipe Pasta (see Index). Place on wax paper, and set aside to be filled later. This can be made a day ahead and stored in refrigerator with wax paper separating crepes.

1½ pounds ground pork
3 cloves garlic, minced
3 teaspoons chili powder
3 tablespoons cider vinegar
1 tablespoon oil
3 tablespoons chopped onion
1 8-ounce can tomato sauce

1 can water
½ teaspoon cumin
6 or 7 drops Tabasco sauce, or to taste
1 teaspoon salt, or to taste
1½ cups shredded Cheddar cheese

Preheat oven to 350°.

In bowl combine ground pork, garlic, 2 teaspoons chili powder, and vinegar.

Heat oil in skillet, and sauté onions on medium heat for 3 or 4 minutes until soft.

Form pork mixture into 1 large ball and place in skillet with onion. As pork is browning, slowly break into small pieces. Cook thoroughly. Pour off all fat. Set aside.

Sauce

In saucepan combine tomato sauce, water, cumin, 1 teaspoon chili powder, Tabasco sauce, and salt. Simmer for ½ hour.

In baking pan 13 by 9 inches, pour ½ cup sauce. Spoon heaping tablespoon of pork mixture on crepe. Top with 1 tablespoon shredded cheese. Fold over and place crepes side by side in baking pan. Repeat until you use all crepes. Pour remaining sauce over all crepes.

Place in 350° oven for 15 minutes. Cover with remaining cheese. Bake for 5 more minutes or until cheese is hot and bubbly.

Total Grams 39.5
Grams per serving 6.6

Noodle Pudding

8 servings

½ pint sour cream
½ pound creamed cottage cheese
¼ cup heavy cream
1 teaspoon salt
1 cup quartered walnuts
3 tablespoons butter, melted

crushed fried pork rinds
½ recipe Pasta (see Index)
2 tablespoon-equivalents brown sugar substitute
½ teaspoon cinnamon

Preheat oven to 375°.

Combine all ingredients except pork rinds, pasta, sugar substitute, and cinnamon. Mix well. Pour into casserole. Top with crushed pork rinds.

Bake in 375° oven for 1½ hours.

Cut pasta into shape of fine noodles. Toss noodles with cooked cheese mixture. Add sugar substitute, cinnamon, and mix. Allow noodle pudding to set in 250° oven for 15 minutes before serving. Top with more crushed pork rinds.

Total Grams   67.0
Grams per serving   8.4

For lovers of noodle pudding only.

VEGETABLES

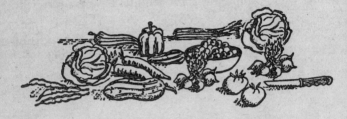

Cauliflower in Butter

6 servings

1 pound cauliflower
5 tablespoons butter
  salt and pepper

(When weighing cauliflower, keep in mind weight of stems and leaves. Judge amount depending on size, so that when cauliflower is broken into flowerets you will have 1 pound.)

Wash cauliflower, removing outer leaves and stem. Remove any bruised parts and break into flowerets.

Steam cauliflower in saucepan, containing 1 inch boiling salted water, for about 10 to 15 minutes. Drain well and place in serving dish.

Melt butter in small saucepan and pour over hot flowerets. Salt and pepper to taste.

Total Grams 24.2
Grams per serving 4.0

Also try it without butter and use Cheese Sauce (see Index).

Cauliflower in Cheese Sauce

6 servings

1 pound cauliflower
1 recipe Cheese Sauce (see Index)

Prepare cauliflower, following directions for Cauliflower in Butter (see Index).

Omit butter and use cheese sauce (3 tablespoons per serving).

Total Grams 36.7
Grams per serving 6.1

Cauliflower Italian Style

6 servings

1 pound cauliflower
½ cup olive oil
½ teaspoon garlic powder
pepper to taste
½ cup grated Parmesan cheese

Wash cauliflower, removing leaves and stem and any bruised portions.

Cook in about 1 inch boiling salted water until barely tender (6 or 7 minutes).

Heat olive oil in saucepan. Add cauliflower and sprinkle with garlic powder. Sauté until lightly browned. Add pepper.

Arrange cauliflower on heated serving dish and sprinkle with Parmesan cheese.

Total Grams 26.1
Grams per serving 4.3

If the aroma doesn't get them, the taste will!

Cauliflower in Hot Dressing

6 servings

2 cups cauliflower,
washed and divided
into flowerets.
3 tablespoons corn or
safflower oil
2 cloves garlic
2 tablespoons onion

1 teaspoon paprika
2 teaspoons vinegar
2 tablespoons water
from cauliflower
¼ teaspoon salt or to
taste

Boil cauliflower in just enough water to cover for 10 to 15 minutes until tender.

In small skillet heat oil and sauté garlic until brown. Remove garlic. Add onion and sauté until soft and transparent. Remove from heat.

Add paprika, vinegar, water, and salt. Mix well and heat.

Pour over drained cauliflower. Cover and simmer for 10 minutes.

Total Grams 28.9
Grams per serving 4.6

Baked Spinach

4 servings

¾ cup spinach (½ frozen
package or 3 cups
fresh)
¼ cup water
3 tablespoons olive oil
3 tablespoons butter
3 tablespoons minced
onion

1 clove garlic, minced
2 slices prosciutto, diced
5 eggs
3 tablespoons cream
pinch of black pepper
3 tablespoons grated
Parmesan cheese

Preheat oven to 350°.

Wash spinach well. Be careful to remove all sand. Do not dry.

Place spinach in saucepan with water, cover, and steam for about 6 minutes. Drain.

Heat olive oil and butter in skillet.

Add onion, garlic, and prosciutto to skillet. Cook slowly until onion is light brown. Add onion mixture to spinach. Simmer for 5 minutes.

Beat eggs with cream, and add pepper. Add spinach mixture and Parmesan cheese to eggs.

Lightly oil an 8-inch-square baking dish. Place mixture in dish, and bake for 30 minutes in 350° oven. Cut into 4 squares.

Total Grams   16.5
Grams per serving   4.5

You'll have no trouble getting people to eat it!

Stuffed Zippy Zucchini

4 servings

2 medium zucchini
3 ounces ricotta cheese
1 teaspoon minced parsley
1 onion, chopped
1 egg white, beaten stiff
1 8-ounce can tomato sauce

Preheat oven to 300°.

Cut zucchini into halves lengthwise and scoop out pulp.

Combine ricotta, parsley, and onion. Mix well. Fold in egg white.

Stuff mixture into halved zucchini. Place in baking dish and pour tomato sauce over top.

Bake in 300° oven for 10 minutes. Lower heat to 250° and cook for 30 more minutes. Baste often.

Total Grams 35.2
Grams per serving 8.8

Vegetable-lover's favorite.

Zesty Zucchini

6 servings

6 small zucchini
4 mushrooms
3 tablespoons olive oil
3 tablespoons diced onion
½ cup grated Parmesan cheese

½ 8-ounce can tomato sauce
1 clove garlic, minced
1 teaspoon mono-sodium glutamate

Preheat oven to 350°.

Wash zucchini. Cut off ends. Slice into ⅛-inch slices. Set aside.

Clean and slice mushrooms.

Heat olive oil in skillet. Add zucchini, mushrooms, and onion. Cover and cook over low heat for 15 minutes, stirring occasionally.

Place zucchini mixture in baking dish. Add ½ Parmesan cheese, tomato sauce, garlic, and monosodium glutamate. Stir with fork.

Sprinkle with remaining cheese.

Bake in 350° oven for 30 minutes.

Total Grams   31.5
Grams per serving   5.2

It will get the vegetable vote!

Zucchini Stuffed with Cream Sauce

6 servings

6 medium zucchini
3 tablespoons mayonnaise
2 tablespoons grated Parmesan cheese
½ cup sliced mushrooms
3 tablespoons olive oil
4 slices lean prosciutto, diced
1 egg yolk
1 teaspoon salt
½ teaspoon pepper
½ teaspoon oregano

Preheat oven to 375°.

In large pot of boiling water, add zucchini and boil for 5 minutes. Remove from heat, and cut zucchini into halves lengthwise. Scoop out pulp and save.

Mix together pulp from zucchini, mayonnaise, Parmesan cheese, mushrooms, prosciutto, egg yolk, salt, pepper, and oregano.

Place zucchini halves in greased baking dish and fill each zucchini half with mixture. Sprinkle with olive oil. Bake in 375° oven for 30 minutes.

Total Grams   29.9
Grams per serving   5.0

This is one of our favorite recipes. Many of our friends ask for it.

String Beans Amandine

4 servings

1 pound fresh or frozen string beans
½ pound mushrooms, sliced
4 tablespoons butter
½ teaspoon seasoned salt
¼ cup slivered almonds

Prepare string beans for cooking. Simmer in small amount of water for 10 minutes. In skillet sauté mushrooms in butter until brown. Add salt and almonds.

Add string beans to skillet. Toss well. Simmer for 4 minutes. Correct seasoning to taste.

Total Grams 48.0
Grams per serving 12.0

Everybody's vegetable favorite!

Green Beans Oregano

6 servings

2 tablespoons oil
2 tablespoons chopped onion
1 clove garlic
1 8-ounce can tomato sauce

¼ cup water
¼ teaspoon oregano
1 9-ounce package frozen green beans
1 pound fresh green beans

Heat oil in saucepan. Lightly brown onion in oil. Add garlic and sauté for 2 minutes. Add tomato sauce, water, and oregano. Simmer for 10 minutes.

Prepare green beans according to directions on package. In last 5 minutes add tomato sauce mixture, cover, and simmer for 10 minutes.

If using fresh beans:

1 pound fresh green beans

Wash and clean beans. Place in saucepan. Add tomato sauce mixture after simmering for 5 minutes. Cover and cook beans slowly for 40 minutes or until tender, and add a little water if necessary.

Total Grams 32.7
Grams per serving 5.4

Mock Potato Dumplings

12 dumplings

½ head cauliflower (1 cup mashed)
2 eggs, beaten
½ cup grated Parmesan cheese

1 teaspoon parsley
1 teaspoon nutmeg
4 tablespoons soya powder
1 tablespoon salt

4 tablespoons butter

Boil cauliflower until soft, for about 25 minutes. Mash with fork or potato masher.

Add eggs, Parmesan cheese, parsley, nutmeg, and soya powder. Shape into walnut-size balls.

Bring large pot of water to rolling boil. Add salt.

Drop cauliflower balls into water. When they rise, remove with slotted spoon.

Heat butter in skillet. Fry balls in skillet until brown on all sides.

Total Grams 45.3
Grams per dumpling 3.1

Serve in soup, as a side dish, or as an hors d'oeuvre.

Eggs and Asparagus with Cream Sauce

6 servings

1 can asparagus tips or 1 pound fresh asparagus, cooked
1 cup mayonnaise
½ cup water
½ cup cream
6 hard-cooked eggs, sliced
paprika

Preheat oven to 350°.

Drain asparagus well and cut each stalk in half.

In saucepan combine mayonnaise, water, and cream. Stir slowly until heated.

In buttered baking dish place layer of sliced eggs, then layer of cream sauce, then layer of asparagus, and finish with layer of egg slices. Top with remaining sauce. Sprinkle top with paprika.

Heat for 10 minutes in 350° oven.

Total Grams 19.3
Grams per serving 3.3

This may also be made and baked in individual oven-proof dishes.

Asparagus with Parmesan Cheese

8 servings

2 pounds fresh asparagus or 3 packages frozen asparagus tips
½ cup butter, melted
½ cup grated Parmesan cheese

Preheat oven to 400°.

Cut tough ends off fresh asparagus. Wash carefully and cook until tender but still firm. (Cook frozen asparagus 2 minutes less than package directs.) Drain well. Arrange in single layer in buttered shallow baking dish. Pour melted butter over asparagus and sprinkle with Parmesan cheese. Bake in 400° oven for 10 minutes, or until lightly browned.

Total Grams   28.4
Grams per serving   3.7

Be careful—do not overcook!

Parsley Onions

6 servings

18 white onions, peeled
  seasoned salt
  sugar substitute
    3 tablespoons parsley

1 tablespoon oil
2 tablespoons butter
½ cup chicken broth

Sprinkle onions with small amount of salt and sugar substitute. Put oil and butter in frypan over medium to high heat. Add onions and cook until lightly browned (about 5 minutes). Add chicken broth, cover, and cook over low heat for ½ hour. Stir several times until onions are coated. Garnish with parsley.

Total Grams   39.8
Grams per serving   6.6

Chinese Snow Pea Pods

6 servings

2 tablespoons vegetable oil
1 onion, chopped fine
1 clove garlic, chopped fine
½ teaspoon seasoned salt
¼ cup chicken broth

¼ cup sliced water chestnuts
1 6-ounce package frozen pea pods
1 tablespoon soy protein seasoning

Heat oil in heavy skillet. Add onion, garlic, salt, and water chestnuts. Sauté until onion is golden. Add frozen pea pods, soy sauce, and chicken broth. Cover and cook for 5 minutes. Uncover and cook for 5 more minutes.

Total Grams 31.8
Grams per serving 5.3

Eggplant Little Shoes

8 servings

4 medium eggplants
2 tablespoons butter or margarine
4 tablespoons onion
1 clove garlic
1 pound chopped beef or lamb
1 8-ounce can tomato sauce
1 teaspoon cumin

1 teaspoon parsley
1 teaspoon seasoned salt
pepper to taste
1 egg
1 tablespoon water
1 tablespoon lemon juice
¼ cup grated Parmesan cheese

Preheat oven to 350°.

Wash eggplants. Do not peel. Parboil whole eggplants in salted boiling water for 5 minutes. Remove. Cut in half lengthwise. Spoon out center pulp carefully and chop, leaving about 1/4 inch around rim.

Melt butter in saucepan. Add onion and garlic. Sauté for 3 minutes. Add chopped meat and chopped eggplant pulp. Stir. Brown lightly. Add tomato sauce, cumin, parsley, salt, and pepper to taste. Cook over low heat until all liquid is absorbed.

Place eggplants in lightly oiled roasting pan or large casserole dish. Stuff with chopped meat mixture.

Beat egg, water, and lemon juice together. Pour over eggplants. Sprinkle with Parmesan cheese. Bake in 350° oven for 20 minutes until lightly browned.

Total Grams 60.5
Grams per serving 7.5

Eggplant for Eating

3 servings

1 medium eggplant	1/4 teaspoon seasoned salt
bowl of salted water	1/4 cup grated Parmesan
olive oil	cheese
1 egg plus 1 yolk	1/2 cup tomato sauce
1/4 cup heavy cream	1/4 cup grated Swiss
1/4 teaspoon nutmeg	cheese

Preheat oven to 375°.

Peel eggplant. Slice thin and put into bowl of salted water. Soak for at least 10 minutes. Remove from water and pat dry.

Pour about 1/8 inch olive oil into frypan. Sauté eggplant slices in oil until well browned on both sides.

(Add more oil if necessary.) Place eggplant in baking dish.

Beat eggs, heavy cream, nutmeg, salt, and Parmesan cheese together. Pour over eggplant. Bake in 375° oven for ½ hour.

Warm tomato sauce. Pour over eggplant. Sprinkle with Swiss cheese. Place under broiler until cheese melts.

Total Grams 29.0
Grams per serving 9.7

Cheese-Stuffed Eggplant

8 servings

4 medium eggplants
2 medium onions
3 tablespoons butter
3 cups crumbled feta cheese
½ cup grated Parmesan cheese

¼ cup ricotta cheese
1 egg
2 tablespoons chopped parsley
seasoned salt

Preheat oven to 350°.

Slice eggplants in half. Scoop out pulp, chop it, and set aside. Reserve shells. Sauté onions in butter until golden. Add eggplant pulp and continue to sauté for about 5 more minutes. Transfer mixture to bowl and let cool.

Add cheeses to mixture, and beat in egg and parsley. Sprinkle on salt. Stuff mixture back into eggplant shells.

Bake in 350° oven for 40 minutes.

> Total Grams 62.1
> Grams per serving 6.8

Can also be served as a main course.

The Most Delicious Cucumbers

4 servings

4 cucumbers, peeled and seeded
½ tablespoon seasoned salt
½ tablespoon tarragon vinegar
¼ cup butter, melted
1 tablespoon minced dill
1 tablespoon minced chives

1 tablespoon minced onion
¼ cup heavy cream
2 tablespoons minced parsley
grated Parmesan cheese

Preheat oven to 375°.

Slice cucumbers to bite-size pieces. Add salt and vinegar. Allow to stand at room temperature for at least 2 hours. Drain and dry thoroughly with paper towels.

Put cucumbers in casserole with butter, dill, chives, and onion. Bake in 375° oven for 25 minutes.

Remove from oven; add heavy cream. Stir over medium heat for about 5 minutes (do not allow to boil). Cream will thicken. Sprinkle with parsley and small amount of Parmesan cheese.

Serve hot.

> Total Grams 24.7
> Grams per serving 6.2

Crazy, creamy, cheesy cucumbers!

Crazy Cabbage

8 servings

1 cabbage, trimmed	¼ cup chopped parsley
1 onion, chopped	1 egg
¼ pound bacon	1 tablespoon grated
2 garlic cloves	Parmesan cheese
2 tablespoons olive oil	seasoned salt
1 cup chicken broth	

Preheat oven to 375°.

Boil cabbage in salted water for 15 minutes. Remove and run under cold water. Core cabbage, leaving outer leaves intact. Chop core and inner leaves. Sauté cabbage, onion, bacon, and garlic together in olive oil.

Mix parsley with egg and Parmesan cheese. Beat well.

Mix egg mixture into sautéed cabbage.

Line deep casserole with aluminum foil. Place large outer cabbage leaves in casserole. Fill middle with sautéed mixture. Pour chicken broth over mixture.

Cover and bake in 375° oven for 1 hour. Remove cover and bake for 30 more minutes.

Remove from casserole by lifting foil out. Serve.

Total Grams 37.8
Grams per serving 4.7

Mushroom Pancakes

2 servings

Prepare as in Hungarian Ham Pancakes (see Index), replacing ham with ½ pound mushrooms.

Total Grams 16.0
Grams per serving 8.0

Ratatouille

12 servings (½-cup servings)

4½ tablespoons olive oil
3 medium zucchini,
    unpeeled,
    quartered, cut into
    1-inch lengths
½ medium eggplant,
    unpeeled, cut into
    1½-inch cubes
salt and pepper to
    taste
2 medium onions,
    chopped

5 cloves garlic, finely
    minced
2 green peppers,
    chopped
1 8-ounce can tomato
    sauce
½ teaspoon thyme
1 teaspoon basil
¼ cup finely chopped
    parsley
lemon wedges

Heat 2½ tablespoons olive oil in large skillet, add zucchini, eggplant, and salt and pepper to taste. Cook, stirring occasionally, for about 10 minutes.

Heat 2 remaining tablespoons olive oil in another skillet. Add onions, garlic, and peppers, and cook until lightly browned. Add tomato sauce and simmer, stirring occasionally, for about 10 minutes.

Add zucchini and eggplant mixtures, then thyme, basil, and parsley. Pour in casserole, cover, and bake in 350° oven for about 20 minutes, or until vegetables are tender.

Can also be served cold with lemon wedges.

Total Grams   48.6
Grams per serving   4.0

This is so tasty it is a good idea to keep it available in the refrigerator for those between-meal snacks.

SAUCES FOR MEAT, POULTRY, FISH, PASTA, VEGETABLES, AND DESSERTS

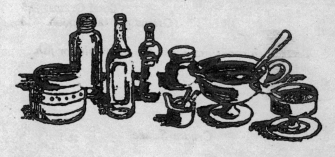

Quick Cream Sauce

16 tablespoons

½ cup mayonnaise
¼ cup water
¼ cup cream

Place all ingredients in saucepan. Heat slowly, stirring constantly, until smooth.

Total Grams   4.6
Grams per tablespoon   .3

Serve with cooked or uncooked vegetables or fish.

Cream Sauce

24 tablespoons

¼ pound sweet butter
3 egg yolks
¼ cup water
¼ cup heavy cream
dash of nutmeg

Place butter in top of double boiler over hot (not boiling) water. Add egg yolks one at a time. Beat constantly with rotary or hand electric beater. Add water and heavy cream. Continue to beat until sauce thickens, about 7 to 10 minutes. Add nutmeg as garnish.

Total Grams   4.1
Grams per tablespoon   Trace

Serve it with Cannelloni with Chicken (see Index).

Bacon Cream Sauce

1½ cups

5 strips bacon
3 tablespoons minced
onion
½ cup mayonnaise
¼ cup heavy cream
2 hard-cooked eggs,
chopped
1 tablespoon lemon
juice

½ teaspoon Dijon
mustard
¼ teaspoon-equivalent
sugar substitute
¼ teaspoon thyme
¼ teaspoon ground
pepper

Fry bacon in large skillet until crisp. Set bacon aside on absorbent paper. Remove skillet from heat.

Pour off all but 2 tablespoons bacon fat. Allow pan to cool.

Add onion, mayonnaise, heavy cream, eggs, lemon juice, mustard, sugar substitute, thyme, and pepper to skillet. Mix well. Crumble bacon into mixture and stir well.

Chill for several hours.

Total Grams 14.2
Grams per tablespoon .6

Serve as a dressing for hot or cold vegetables. Good with raw vegetables too.

Frozen Horseradish Cream

19 tablespoons

1 cup heavy cream
2 tablespoons white horseradish
1 teaspoon seasoned salt
2 teaspoons Dijon mustard

Whip heavy cream until stiff.

Mix together horseradish, salt, and mustard. Carefully fold mixture into whipped cream. Freeze until firm.

Total Grams   11.3
Grams per serving   .6

Adds a zesty flavor—use with Short Ribs in Rich Beef Broth (see Index).

Avocado Cream Sauce

12 tablespoons

2 tablespoons mayon-
  naise
pinch of garlic powder
1 minced anchovy fillet
4 tablespoons sour
  cream

½ teaspoon lemon juice
½ California avocado
½ teaspoon seasoned salt
½ teaspoon Blue Cheese
  seasoning
2 thin slices boiled ham

Place all ingredients in blender container. Blend at medium speed until smooth. (If it seems too thick, add a little water.)

Refrigerate for at least 1 hour.

Serve with meats or vegetables.

Total Grams   10.8
Grams per tablespoon   .9

It's a real flavor enhancer.

Hollandaise Sauce

1½ cups

2 tablespoons tarragon
vinegar
½ teaspoon seasoned salt
1 tablespoon cold water
4 egg yolks

2 sticks butter, at room
temperature
1 teaspoon lemon juice
1 tablespoon heavy
cream

Combine vinegar and salt in saucepan and cook rapidly to reduce to half. Remove from heat and add water. Place yolks in saucepan and beat with wire whisk until creamy. Place pan over double boiler and begin to add butter a little at a time. Beat with whisk as butter is melting.

When sauce is thick, add lemon juice and heavy cream. Beat again. Keep warm until ready to serve.

Total Grams 5.3

Cheese Sauce

18 tablespoons

¾ cup cream
⅓ cup water
¾ pound (1½ cups) Cheddar cheese, diced
1 teaspoon mustard
1 teaspoon salt
½ teaspoon paprika

In double boiler combine ingredients for cheese sauce. Simmer slowly. Stir constantly until smooth.

Total Grams 12.5
Grams per tablespoon .6

Try it with Cauliflower in Butter and Eggs Florentine (see Index).

Tartare Sauce

16 tablespoons

¾ cup mayonnaise
1 tablespoon tarragon
    vinegar
1 teaspoon finely
    chopped onion
1 teaspoon capers

1 teaspoon finely
    chopped pickles
1 teaspoon finely
    chopped olives
1 teaspoon finely
    chopped parsley

Combine all ingredients. Mix well.

Store in covered jar in refrigerator. Will keep for several weeks.

Total Grams 4.6
Grams per tablespoon .3

Cocktail Sauce

1 cup

1 8-ounce can tomato sauce
1 tablespoon horseradish
1 teaspoon Worcestershire sauce
1 teaspoon lemon juice

Mix all ingredients. Chill thoroughly.

Total Grams 18.4
Grams per tablespoon 1.2

Mornay Sauce

20 tablespoons

2 tablespoons butter
½ teaspoon seasoned salt
or salt
dash of cayenne
pepper
¼ teaspoon dry mustard
½ teaspoon Dijon
mustard

1 cup heavy cream
¼ cup grated Parmesan
cheese
2 tablespoons mayon-
naise

Melt butter. Add salt, pepper, dry mustard, and Dijon mustard.

Remove from fire. Mix in heavy cream.

Stir over low flame just until it comes to boil (do not boil). Add Parmesan cheese and mayonnaise. Simmer for 2 minutes.

Serve hot.

Total Grams 9.6
Grams per serving .5

Mushroom Sauce

26 tablespoons

2 tablespoons butter
½ cup mushrooms
2 teaspoons diced onion
1 recipe Quick Cream Sauce (see Index)

Melt butter in skillet. Sauté mushrooms and onion in butter until soft and light brown.

Fold into cream sauce. Simmer for 5 minutes.

> Total Grams   10.6
> Grams per tablespoon   .4

Try it with Taste Delight Pancakes (see Index).

Parsley Butter Sauce

4 servings

4 sprigs parsley, chopped (tops only)
1 small clove garlic, chopped fine
¼ pound sweet butter, melted
¼ teaspoon Worcestershire sauce

Add parsley and garlic to melted butter. Cook for 1 minute over medium flame. Add Worcestershire sauce.

Serve immediately.

(If you must reheat this sauce, use very low flame.)

> Total Grams   3.6
> Grams per serving (2 tablespoons)   .9

Serve it with Stuffed Steak (see Index).

Pasta Sauce

14 servings (½ cup each)

2 pork chops
5 tablespoons olive oil
6 8-ounce cans tomato sauce
3 8-ounce cans water
3 large cloves garlic, minced
1 teaspoon salt
1 pound sweet or hot Italian sausages
1 pound ground chuck
1 teaspoon oregano
1 teaspoon thyme
2 teaspoon-equivalents sugar substitute (or to taste)

Place pork chops and 2 tablespoons olive oil in large heavy pot. Brown chops well. Add tomato sauce, water, garlic, and salt.

Bring to slow boil. Allow to boil.

Place sausages in heavy skillet without any oil. Prick sausages with fork. Cook until well browned on all sides. Slice into one-half-inch pieces. Drain well and discard drippings. Add to pork chop mixture.

Put ground chuck in skillet with 3 tablespoons olive oil. Keep in large ball and as it browns break up slowly. (This is done to allow meat to retain its juices.) When meat is lightly browned, add to pork chop mixture.

Simmer for 3 hours, stirring occasionally.

Add oregano and thyme the last ½ hour. When mixture is finished cooking, add sugar substitute.

Total Grams 82.8
Grams per serving 5.9

*Keep this on hand in the freezer.
You'll use it a lot.*

Curry Cumin Sauce

2 cups

1 cup mayonnaise
½ cup water
½ cup cream
1 teaspoon curry powder
(or to taste)

1 teaspoon cumin (or to taste)
½ teaspoon cayenne

Heat all ingredients in saucepan. Stir until smooth.
Taste for curry flavor. Adjust if necessary.

Total Grams   11.1

Doubles the flavor of everything you use it with.

Green Sauce for Pasta

6 servings

5 cloves garlic, minced
2 tablespoons dried basil
¼ teaspoon thyme
¼ cup grated Parmesan
  cheese
4 tablespoons chopped
  walnuts

6 tablespoons olive oil
6 tablespoons butter
2 tablespoons chopped
  parsley

Place garlic, basil, thyme, Parmesan cheese, walnuts,
and 2 tablespoons oil in blender. Blend until smooth.
Add remaining oil, 2 tablespoons at a time, and blend.

Serve on pasta topped with 1 tablespoon butter per
serving.

Total Grams   12.1
Grams per serving   2.0

Mustard Sauce

20 tablespoons

4 tablespoons Dijon mustard
1 cup sour cream
2 tablespoons chopped chives

Mix ingredients well. Refrigerate.

Total Grams   14.9
Grams per serving   .8

*Serve with Fresh Spring Salmon Mousse or
Egg Foo Yung (see Index).*

Chocolate Sauce

8 tablespoons

1 square unsweetened chocolate
½ cup cream
1 teaspoon-equivalent sugar substitute
1½ teaspoons vanilla

In small saucepan place chocolate and cream. Warm
slowly, but do not boil. Stir constantly until chocolate
melts.

Remove from heat, and add sugar substitute and
vanilla.

Total Grams   14.9
Grams per serving   1.8

Poppy Seed Dessert Dressing

22 tablespoons

2 teaspoons poppy seeds
  pinch of onion powder
½ cup olive oil
½ cup vegetable oil
⅓ cup white vinegar
2 tablespoons Cointreau

Beat all ingredients together.

> Total Grams 13.0
> Grams per tablespoon .6

*To dress up desserts, for example, Cottage Cheese and
Fruit (see Index).*

Strawberry Sauce

> 18 tablespoons

2 cups strawberries (fresh or frozen unsweetened)
2 tablespoons kirschwasser liqueur

Mash strawberries with fork. Pour liqueur on strawberries. Mix well and chill.

> Total Grams 39.0
> Grams per serving 2.2

Serve with ice cream or whole strawberries.

SALADS AND SALAD DRESSINGS

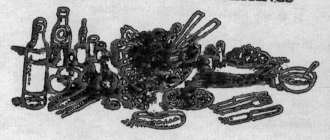

Shrimp Deviled Eggs from the Sea

6 servings

6 hard-cooked eggs, prepared for stuffing (see Index)
1 pound fresh shrimp or 2 to 4 1-ounce cans, minced
½ teaspoon salt

½ teaspoon dry mustard
2 tablespoons mayonnaise
1 recipe Curry Sauce (see Index)
4 scrambled eggs (see Index)

Prepare hard-cooked eggs.

Preheat oven to 350°.

Mix yolks with 6 tablespoons shrimp, salt, mustard, and mayonnaise. Place mixture in egg whites.

Make curry sauce.

Make scrambled eggs.

Spoon layer of curry sauce in pretty casserole dish. Add layer of scrambled eggs.

Place deviled eggs on top of scrambled eggs. Place shrimp between each egg.

Pour remaining sauce on top.

Heat in moderate 350° over for 20 minutes.

Total Grams 24.7
Grams per serving 4.1

Try it with chopped leftover chicken.

Tuna Delight

Makes 1 cup

1 7-ounce can tuna, drained
2 3-ounce packages cream cheese, at room temperature
1 or 2 stalks celery, finely chopped
¼ cup mayonnaise
1 teaspoon seasoned salt

Combine all ingredients, mixing well. Chill.

To stuff celery or use between lettuce leaves.

Total Grams   7.4

Tuna Surprise

2 servings

½ cup whipped cream cheese
2 tablespoons heavy cream
1 13-ounce can tuna fish
1 tablespoon white horseradish

1 teaspoon tarragon
salt and pepper to taste
6 slices Nova Scotia smoked salmon
lettuce, chopped
lemon wedges

Combine cream cheese and heavy cream in bowl. Add tuna fish (broken into small pieces), horseradish, tarragon, salt, and pepper.

Spread mixture on slices of smoked salmon.

Roll smoked salmon up, toothpick it, and place on bed of chopped lettuce. Garnish with lemon wedges.

Total Grams   6.2
Grams per serving   3.1

The taste is the real surprise!

Salmon Salad in a Hurry

1 serving

1 7-ounce can salmon
2 chopped scallions
½ stalk diced celery
3 tablespoons Roquefort dressing (see Index)

Remove bone and skin of salmon. Break in chunks in bowl. Mix scallions and celery with salmon. Turn into salad bowl and pour dressing over. This can also be served on lettuce leaves.

Total Grams 2.6

Chicken Salad Ham Rolls

4 servings

1 cup cooked chicken
   diced
¼ cup mayonnaise
¼ cup chopped parsley
¼ cup chopped celery
   leaves

1 teaspoon seasoned salt
6 black olives, diced
4 tablespoons minced
   fresh green pepper
8 slices boiled ham
lettuce leaves

Combine all ingredients except ham and lettuce.

Spread mixture on ham slices and roll each one up, toothpick it, and place it seam side down on bed of lettuce leaves.

Total Grams 16.6
Grams per serving 4.2

They'll eat them up as fast as you can roll them up!

Chicken Salad in the Round

3 servings

1 cup minced leftover
chicken
6 tablespoons mayon-
naise
2 tablespoons Dijon
mustard
¼ cup chopped parsley

¼ cup chopped celery
1 teaspoon seasoned salt
6 slices boiled ham
¼ head of lettuce,
chopped
green pepper rings

Place chicken in bowl. Mix mayonnaise and mustard together and add to chicken. Add parsley, celery, and salt. Mix well. Spread mixture on ham slices, roll slices up, and toothpick them.

Place on bed of lettuce with seam side down. Garnish with green pepper rings.

Total Grams 16.4
Grams per serving 5.5

Ham Salad Donna

8 servings

¾ pound lean ham, diced
½ large green pepper,
diced
4 stalks celery, diced
½ cup coarsely chopped
walnuts
¼ cup sour cream

¼ cup mayonnaise
½ teaspoon curry powder
½ teaspoon lemon juice
½ teaspoon soy protein
seasoning
1 cantaloupe
8 parsley sprigs

Combine ham, pepper, celery, and walnuts. Add sour cream, mayonnaise, curry powder, lemon juice, and soy sauce in that order. Refrigerate.

Discard seeds and skin of cantaloupe and slice to form 8 rings.

Lay cantaloupe ring on plate. Fill center of ring with ham salad. Garnish with parsley sprig.

Total Grams 34.1
Grams per serving 4.3

A really beautiful salad!

Roast Beef Salad

2 servings

1 cup leftover roast beef, cut into strips
½ cup sour cream
1 teaspoon Worcestershire sauce
2 teaspoons diced green pepper
1 teaspoon chopped pimento
1 teaspoon chopped black olives

Mix ingredients together thoroughly.

Total Grams 6.0
Grams per serving 3.0

Luscious leftovers!

Bacon and Egg Salad

6 servings

9 hard-cooked eggs
9 slices bacon, cooked crisp
½ teaspoon seasoned salt
¼ teaspoon dry mustard
¼ cup mayonnaise

Chop eggs and bacon together in wooden chopping bowl. Add salt and mustard.

Fold in mayonnaise and mix well.

Total Grams 8.6
Grams per serving 1.5

A variation on an old favorite!

Eggplant Relish

46 tablespoons (23 1-ounce servings)

1 eggplant
1 green pepper
1 onion
3 tablespoons olive oil
2 tablespoons wine vinegar
salt and pepper to taste

Boil eggplant until soft. Drain well. Peel, slice, and dry. Chop eggplant with pepper and onion until all vegetables are chopped very fine. Add olive oil and vinegar. Mix well. Season to taste.

Refrigerate.

Total Grams 32.3
Grams per serving 1.4

Serve as a garnish with meat, fish, or egg dishes.

Radish Relish

8 servings (2 cups)

40 radishes
 water
 2 teaspoons seasoned salt
½ cup sour cream
 1 tablespoon vinegar
 1 tablespoon minced chives

Place radishes in blender and add enough water to just cover them. Blend at medium speed until radishes are chopped up (for about 6 seconds).

Put radishes in strainer and allow to drain well for about ½ hour.

Place radishes in bowl, and add salt, sour cream, vinegar, and chives.

Refrigerate.

Total Grams 23.2
Grams per serving 3.0

Celery Salad

8 servings

6 celery stalks, chopped
 1 large onion, chopped
¾ cup mayonnaise
¼ cup sour cream
½ cup Dijon mustard
 seasoned salt
 1 teaspoon poppy seeds

Place celery and onion in bowl. Mix in mayonnaise and sour cream.

Add mustard, salt, and poppy seeds.

Chill until ready to serve. Serve on lettuce.

> Total Grams 34.6
> Grams per serving 4.4

Creamy and chewy—and tasty!

Mushroom Salad

6 servings

8 slices bacon, diced
1 small onion, minced
2 tablespoons butter,
melted
3 tablespoons lemon juice

2 tablespoons parsley
1 pound white mush-
rooms, thinly sliced
grated Parmesan cheese

Fry bacon until transparent. Add minced onion; continue frying until bacon is crisp and onion is golden. Pour off bacon fat.

Add butter, lemon juice, and parsley. Bring to boil.

Pour over mushrooms, and garnish with Parmesan cheese to taste.

> Total Grams 29.3
> Grams per serving .5

A real go-along for any meal.

Spinach Salad Special

4 servings

1 pound fresh spinach
1 7-ounce can tuna, crumbled
¼ pound bacon, cooked crisp and broken into small
  pieces.
¼ cup grated Parmesan cheese
1½ recipes Dressing of the House (see Index)

Wash spinach carefully to remove all sand. Dry thoroughly. Place spinach in bowl. Add tuna and bacon to spinach. Toss well. Sprinkle with cheese. Pour on salad dressing, and toss again.

Total Grams   26.5
Grams per serving   6.6
Dressing per serving   1.3

An unexpected lunch-munch treat.

Avocado and Spinach Salad

6 servings

1 onion, coarsely
  chopped
2 tablespoons butter
1 10-ounce package
  frozen chopped leaf
  spinach
2 hard-cooked eggs,
  chopped

1 avocado, peeled and
  chopped
½ teaspoon caraway
  seeds
½ cup Vinaigrette Cream
  Dressing (see Index)

Sauté onion in butter until golden.

Cook spinach according to package directions. Drain very well. Add onion, eggs, avocado, and caraway seeds to spinach.

Put in salad bowl and toss well with Vinaigrette Cream Dressing.

Total Grams	31.3
Grams per serving	5.3
Vinaigrette Cream Dressing (per tablespoon)	.3

Looks as pretty as it tastes good!

Seafood and Avocado Salad

6 servings

1 large avocado, pitted, peeled, and cubed
1½ pounds crabmeat or tuna fish
2 stalks celery, chopped
6 radishes sliced
4 tablespoons lemon juice

4 tablespoons tarragon vinegar
½ small onion, chopped
¼ teaspoon cayenne pepper
seasoned salt to taste

Toss all ingredients together well.

Serve with Thousand Island Dressing (see Index).

Total Grams	29.5
Grams per serving	5.0

Impressive (and expensive) as well as delicious!

Crab-Stuffed Avocado

4 servings

½ cup mayonnaise
½ cup minced celery
¼ cup minced pimento
2 teaspoons lemon juice
dash of Tabasco
sauce
⅛ teaspoon Worcester-
shire sauce

2 ripe avocados
salt
crisp salad greens
1½ cups chilled cooked
or canned crab-
meat or lobster

Combine mayonnaise, celery, pimento, lemon juice, Tabasco and Worcestershire sauces to make dressing.

Sprinkle halved avocados with a little more lemon juice and salt. Arrange each half on salad greens.

Fill halves with crabmeat. Top with dressing.

Total Grams 43.2
Grams per serving 10.8

A luncheon specialty!

Cole Slaw Our Way

6 servings (½ cup)

¼ cup Dijon mustard
¼ cup mayonnaise
½ teaspoon-equivalent sugar substitute
1 tablespoon lemon juice
½ teaspoon salt
1 medium cabbage, shredded (3 cups)

Mix mustard, mayonnaise, sugar substitute, lemon juice, and salt together. Add cabbage and toss well.

Total Grams 41.4
Grams per serving 7.0

You'll decide it's your way too!

Cottage Cheese Lime Mold

6 servings

1 envelope sugar-free
  lime gelatin
½ cup mayonnaise
½ cup sour cream
1 teaspoon lemon juice
1 pound cottage cheese
  (2 cups)

½ cantaloupe, finely
  diced
sugar substitute to
  taste

Prepare gelatin according to package directions, but do not add cold water.

Add mayonnaise, sour cream, and lemon juice to gelatin. Beat with hand electric beater or rotary beater.

Fold in cottage cheese and cantaloupe. Test for sweetness.

Pour into wet 1-quart mold. Rerfrigerate for at least 2 hours before serving.

Total Grams 37.6
Grams per serving 6.3

Pretty special!

Fruity Cottage Cheese Salad

6 servings

½ teaspoon salt
1 teaspoon grated lemon
  rind
2 tablespoons lemon
  juice
1 tablespoon grated
  orange rind

2 cups creamed cottage
  cheese
1 head lettuce
½ cup sliced strawberries
  (1 cup whole)

Combine salt, lemon rind, lemon juice, orange rind, and cottage cheese.

Wash and dry crisp lettuce. Arrange on plate. Turn out cottage cheese, and surround with strawberries.

Total Grams 39.8
Grams per serving 6.6

Cottage cheese never tasted so good!

A Mold of Roquefort

12 servings

1 envelope unflavored
  gelatin
¼ cup cold water
6 ounces Roquefort
  cheese
6 ounces cream cheese,
  softened

½ cup heavy cream
4 scallions minced
2 tablespoons pine nuts
4 black olives, chopped
  seasoned salt to taste

Sprinkle gelatin into water. Push Roquefort cheese through strainer. Add cream cheese and heavy cream to Roquefort cheese. Mix well. Add gelatin, scallions, pine nuts, olives, and salt to cheese mixtures.

Pour into 3-cup ring mold that has been sprayed with grease substitute. Chill. Occasionally stir gently until set.

Total Grams 17.1
Grams per serving 1.4

Roquefort cheese lovers will eat it with everything.

Mock Potato Salad

8 servings (½ cup)

1 medium rutabaga
  pot of boiling water
½ teaspoon-equivalent
  sugar substitute
1 tablespoon lemon
  juice
½ cup finely chopped
  scallions
1 medium dill pickle,
  chopped

1 cup minced celery
  with leaves
1½ teaspoons salt
  dash of paprika
¾ cup mayonnaise
4 hard-cooked eggs,
  chopped

Pare rutabaga, and cut into 4 pieces. Drop into boiling water. Continue to boil until tender (about ½ hour). Drain well. Cool.

After rutabaga has cooled, dice (should be approximately 2½ cups), and place in salad bowl. Sprinkle with sugar substitute and lemon juice. Add scallions, pickle, celery, salt, paprika, and mayonnaise to rutabaga.

Toss well. Fold in eggs. Chill before serving.

Total Grams 69.4
Grams per serving 8.7

For those of us who love potato salad—and even for those who hate it!

Tossed Salad with Tomato Dressing

12 servings

2 heads lettuce (your choice)
2 tomatoes
6 scallions (green onions)
1 tablespoon dry mustard
½ teaspoon garlic powder
1 tablespoon Dijon mustard
1 teaspoon seasoned salt
2 tablespoons olive oil
2 tablespoons tarragon vinegar
4 tablespoons vegetable oil
1 tablespoon mayonnaise

Wash lettuce, dry thoroughly, and break into bite-size pieces. Refrigerate.

Tomato dressing
Chop tomatoes and scallions together until puréed. Add all other ingredients except lettuce. Beat with wire whisk. Refrigerate.

When ready to serve, place lettuce in large salad bowl, pour dressing on top, and toss well. Serve immediately.

Total Grams 42.5
Grams per serving 3.5

Very basic—goes with everything.

Green Bean Salad

6 servings

1 pound fresh green beans
½ cup water
⅓ cup wine vinegar
½ cup olive oil
½ teaspoon salt
½ teaspoon pepper
3 tablespoons thinly sliced onion
2 cloves garlic, diced fine
½ teaspoon oregano
1 teaspoon parsley

Wash and break off ends of beans. Place in saucepan with water. Simmer for about 10 minutes. Reserve ⅛ cup water and drain rest.

Combine water, vinegar, oil, salt, pepper, onion, garlic, oregano, and parsley.

Pour over beans. Store in covered container. Chill overnight.

Total Grams   40.3
Grams per serving   6.4

Make plenty—everybody loves it!

Not Just Another Tossed Salad

12 servings

½ pound fresh spinach, washed and dried
1 small head Boston lettuce, washed and dried
½ 7¼-ounce can large black olives, sliced
½ cup diced celery
5 scallions, diced
6 radishes, sliced
½ cup diced raw cauliflowerets

1 avocado, peeled and diced
8 slices bacon, crisp and crumbled
2 soft-boiled eggs (2 minutes)
½ cup lemon juice
¼ cup peanut oil
¼ cup grated Parmesan cheese
seasoned salt to taste

Break spinach and lettuce into bite-size pieces.

Toss all vegetables and bacon together in bowl.

Make dressing by beating eggs, lemon juice, oil, cheese, and salt together.

Pour over vegetables and serve.

Total Grams 51.7
Grams per serving 4.3

Serve with any and all of your meat favorites!

Greek Salad

6 servings

1 large tomato, cubed (in bite-size pieces)	2 tablespoons capers
½ large green pepper, cubed	¼ pound feta cheese, crumbled
½ large cucumber, pared and cubed	12 thin slices pepperoni
	4 tablespoons olive oil
½ 6-ounce can ripe pitted olives	2 tablespoons wine vinegar
3 scallions, diced	¼ teaspoon cracked pepper
½ teaspoon oregano	

Combine tomato, pepper, cucumber, olives, scallions, capers, cheese, and pepperoni in salad bowl. Mix olive oil, vinegar, pepper, and oregano together in small bowl. Pour dressing over vegetables. Toss and serve.

Total Grams 25.0
Grams per serving 4.1

A really lovely salad—enhances everything, including appetites!

Sauerkraut Salad

6 servings

1 pound sauerkraut
(delicatessen sauer-
kraut, not canned)
2 stalks celery, diced
½ large green pepper,
diced

½ large onion, diced
¾ teaspoon-equivalent
sugar substitute
½ cup olive oil
½ cup wine vinegar

Place sauerkraut in colander. Rinse well with cold water. Drain. Press water from sauerkraut with paper towels.

Add celery, pepper, and onion to dry sauerkraut.

Place sugar substitute, oil, and vinegar in small bowl. Mix together very well.

Pour over sauerkraut and toss.

Refrigerate for 4 to 5 hours. Serve cold.

Total Grams 36.8
Grams per serving 6.1

A salad with a German flavor.

Honeydew and Seafood

6 servings

1 1-pound honeydew
melon
1 6½-ounce can tuna
fish
1 4½-ounce can shrimp
1 medium cucumber,
peeled and cubed

½ pound raw mush-
rooms, sliced
½ cup mayonnaise
2 tablespoons tomato
sauce
½ teaspoon seasoned salt

Cut melon in half lengthwise. Scoop out center and make balls. Leave rim ¼ inch wide. Cut into thirds.

In bowl combine tuna fish, shrimp (save a few for garnish), cucumber, mushrooms, and melon balls.

Combine mayonnaise, tomato sauce, and salt. Pour dressing over seafood. Mix well.

Fill melon shells. Garnish with some shrimp.

If you prefer low fat, eliminate dressing, and use juice of 1 lemon.

Total Grams 44.4
Grams per serving 7.3

Our Favorite Roquefort Dressing

1 cup

¼ cup tarragon vinegar
¼ teaspoon seasoned salt
3 turns of pepper mill
6 tablespoons olive oil

2 tablespoons heavy cream
½ teaspoon lemon juice
¼ cup crumbled Roquefort cheese

Beat all ingredients together except cheese. Stir in cheese.

Total Grams 6.7

Basic French Dressing

½ cup

3 tablespoons tarragon
    vinegar
1 tablespoon lemon
    juice
½ teaspoon seasoned salt
3 turns of pepper mill

6 tablespoons olive oil
2 tablespoons vegetable
    oil
½ teaspoon Dijon
    mustard
¼ teaspoon dry mustard

Beat all ingredients together until well blended.

Total Grams 2.5

Sherry Dressing

32 tablespoons

½ cup white wine vinegar
¼ teaspoon white pepper
1½ cups olive oil
⅓ cup sherry
2 tablespoons chopped parsley
⅛ teaspoon sugar substitute

Thoroughly combine vinegar and pepper. Add olive
oil, and beat with fork until well mixed. Beat in remaining ingredients. Chill.

Total Grams 11.3
Grams per tablespoon .4

Delicious on cold vegetables or fruit.

Cucumber Dressing

28 tablespoons (1¾ cups)

1 cup sour cream
¼ cup tarragon vinegar
½ cup finely diced cucumber
1 teaspoon salt
¼ teaspoon-equivalent sugar substitute
dash of paprika

Place all ingredients in blender. Cover. Blend until smooth.

Total Grams 16.7
Grams per tablespoon .6

Really dresses up a salad!

Sour Cream Dressing

19 tablespoons

1 cup sour cream
1 teaspoon dillweed
1 tablespoon wine vinegar
½ teaspoon salt
2 tablespoons finely chopped green pepper

Beat sour cream until smooth. Add remaining ingredients and mix well.

Total Grams 14.0
Grams per tablespoon .8

For a really smooth salad.

Russian Dressing

20 tablespoons

½ cup mayonnaise
½ cup sour cream
1 tablespoon Dijon
    mustard
1 tablespoon Worcester-
    shire sauce

2 tablespoons tomato
    sauce
½ teaspoon grated onion
⅛ teaspoon garlic powder

Combine ingredients. Mix well.

Total Grams 9.7
Grams per tablespoon .5

It has a kick to it!

Vinaigrette Cream Dressing

32 tablespoons

½ cup tarragon vinegar
¾ teaspoon salt
¼ teaspoon cracked
    pepper
1½ cups olive oil (or ½
    cup olive oil and
    1 cup vegetable
    oil)
1 teaspoon chopped
    green olives

1 teaspoon chopped
    parsley
3 tablespoons sour
    cream
1 yolk from hard-
    cooked egg, finely
    chopped

Mix vinegar, salt, and pepper. Add oil, olives, parsley,
sour cream, and chopped yolk.

Beat well with fork. Chill for several hours.

Total Grams 8.2
Grams per tablespoon .3

Serve with Avocado and Spinach Salad (see Index).

Dressing of the House

Enough for 2 cups of greens

2 tablespoons olive oil
4 tablespoons vegetable oil
2 tablespoons tarragon vinegar
1 teaspoon seasoned salt

1 teaspoon Dijon mustard
1/4 teaspoon garlic
1 tablespoon mayonnaise
1/4 teaspoon sugar substitute

Put all ingredients in screw-top jar. Close jar and shake until everything is well blended. Refrigerate.

Total Grams 3.5

Will last a long time in the refrigerator.

Thousand Island Dressing

22 servings (1 ounce)

6 scallions (green onions)
1 kosher dill pickle
2 tomatoes
1/2 teaspoon garlic powder

1 teaspoon seasoned salt
2 tablespoons olive oil
2 tablespoons tarragon vinegar
2 tablespoons mayonnaise

Chop scallions, pickle, and tomatoes together in wooden chopping bowl. Add rest of ingredients and mix well. Refrigerate.

Total Grams   22.1

Avocado Dressing

24 tablespoons

1 ripe medium avocado, cubed
½ cup lemon juice
¼ cup mayonnaise
1 teaspoon-equivalent sugar substitute
¼ teaspoon salt
¼ teaspoon paprika

Blend all ingredients at high speed until smooth.

Total Grams   23.6
Grams per tablespoon   1.0

Green on greens!

DESSERTS

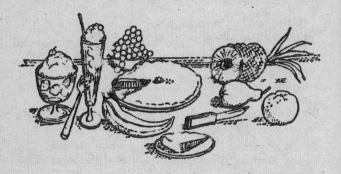

Coconut Cream Pie

10 servings

½ cup coconut
⅛ cup Cointreau
1 tablespoon butter
2½ cups heavy cream
1 envelope unflavored gelatin
¼ cup cold water
2 tablespoon-

equivalents white sugar substitute
4 egg whites at room temperature
2 teaspoons vanilla
1 Meringue Shell (see Index) (optional)

Place coconut in flameproof bowl. Heat Cointreau and ignite. Pour over coconut. (Flames will be high.)

Heat butter in skillet. Add coconut and lightly toast it.

Remove 2 tablespoons toasted coconut and set aside. Add 1 cup heavy cream to skillet. Simmer.

Sprinkle gelatin over cold water. Mix well. Add to cream. Simmer and stir until it begins to thicken. Remove from heat. Add 1 teaspoon-equivalent sugar substitute. Cool.

Beat egg whites until stiff with 1 tablespoon-equivalent sugar substitute. Fold egg whites into cool cream mixture.

Pour mixture into pie plate sprayed with imitation grease. Refrigerate until firm.

Beat 1½ cups heavy cream with vanilla and 2 teaspoon-equivalent sugar substitute. Pile on top of firm cream mixture. Refrigerate for at least 2 hours before serving. Sprinkle with remaining coconut.

Total Grams 34.5
Grams per serving 3.5

One of those "you-won't-believe-you're-on-a-diet" desserts!

Chocolate Mint Pie

8 servings

½ cup chopped pecans
  or walnuts
1 Meringue Shell (see
  Index)
2 ounces unsweetened
  chocolate
2 tablespoons hot water
2 teaspoons peppermint
  extract

1 teaspoon vanilla
1 tablespoon crème de
  cacao
2 teaspoons brown
  sugar substitute
2 cups cream, whipped
1 teaspoon sugar sub-
  stitute (white)

Preheat oven to 275°.

Sprinkle chopped nuts over meringue shell and bake for 1 hour in 275° oven until lightly browned and crisp to touch. Cool, preferably leaving in oven until cool.

Melt chocolate in double broiler, stir in water, and cook until thickened. Remove from heat, and add peppermint extract, vanilla, crème de cacao, brown sugar substitute, and fold in 1 cup whipped cream that has been mixed with 1 teaspoon white sugar substitute.

Fill meringue shell and chill for 2 to 3 hours.

Just before serving, spread remaining 1 cup whipped cream over top.

Total Grams   45.0
Grams per serving   5.6

Delicious! Worth a little extra time and effort!

Italian Sponge Cake

8 servings

5 eggs, separated, at
    room temperature
3 tablespoon-equivalents
    sugar substitute
1 tablespoon and 1 tea-
    spoon vanilla
½ teaspoon grated lemon
    rind

3 tablespoons soya
    powder
4 tablespoons heavy
    cream
½ teaspoon cream of
    tartar

Preheat oven to 325°.

Spray a layer cake pan with imitation grease.

Place egg yolks and sugar substitute in bowl. Beat with electric *hand* mixer until well blended. Add vanilla and lemon rind. Continue to beat and add soya powder 1 tablespoon at a time. Beat until well blended. Add heavy cream.

Beat egg whites with cream of tartar until stiff. Fold yolk mixture into whites with an under and over movement. Be careful not to break down egg whites.

Turn into layer cake pan and bake in 325° oven until done (about ½ hour).

Total Grams   23.7
Grams per serving   3.0

A real snack favorite with coffee!

Strawberry Torte

8 servings

        6 egg whites
        1 tablespoon-equivalent sugar substitute
        1 cup heavy cream
        1 teaspoon vanilla
        2 packages sugar-free strawberry gelatin
    1½ cups strawberries

Preheat oven to 275°

Beat egg whites until foamy. Add sugar substitute. Beat until stiff. Spray a 10-inch pie plate with imitation grease. Spread egg whites to form pie shell Bake in 275° oven for 1 hour. Open oven door and leave shell in for 1½ more hours.

Whip heavy cream with vanilla. Add gelatin.

Slice all but 8 large strawberries. Fold sliced strawberries into cream. Chill well. Just before serving, pile strawberry mixture into pie shell.

Garnish with whole strawberries.

                        Total Grams   38.7
                    Grams per serving   4.8

Delicate preparation is the secret!

Coffee Cream Layer Cake

10 servings

5 eggs, separated, at
   room temperature
5 teaspoon-equivalents
   brown sugar sub-
   stitute
2 cups heavy cream
1½ teaspoons instant
   coffee

½ tablespoon gelatin
1 tablespoon cold water
3 tablespoons butter,
   at room tem-
   perature
2 teaspoons mocha
   extract
½ cup chopped walnuts

Preheat oven to 275°.

Spray 3 round layer cake pans with imitation grease.

Beat egg whites until they form soft peaks. Add 1 tea-spoon brown sugar substitute and beat until stiff. Divide among three pans. Bake in 275° oven for 45 minutes.

Combine 1 cup heavy cream and instant coffee in top of double boiler. Stir with wire whisk until powder dissolves. Dissolve gelatin in cold water. Add gelatin to coffee mixture and heat just to boiling. Stir constantly with whisk. Remove from heat. Beat in 4 egg yolks, 1 yolk at a time. Add butter and beat well until dissolved. Add extract and remaining sugar substitute. Put in freezer to cool.

Whip remaining cup heavy cream until stiff.

When coffee mixture is cool, fold into whipped cream and refrigerate until layers are cooked and cooled. Pile cream between layers of meringue as you would frost a layer cake. Top with cream, making sure to cover sides.

Sprinkle nuts on top and sides. Refrigerate until serving time.

Total Grams   35.0
Grams per serving   3.5

It's extra rich—extra special!

Sweet Crepes

8 servings

1 cup cottage cheese	1 cup and 3 table-
6 eggs	spoons heavy
3 tablespoons soya	cream
powder	2½ teaspoon-equivalents
6 tablespoons vegetable	sugar substitute
oil	1 teaspoon vanilla
½ cup brandy	

Place cottage cheese, eggs, soya powder, 3 tablespoons vegetable oil, 3 tablespoons heavy cream, and 1½ teaspoons sugar substitute in blender. Blend until smooth.

Place 3 remaining tablespoons vegetable oil in crepe pan. Allow to get very hot. Put enough of crepe mixture in pan to just cover bottom. Brown on one side, turn and brown on other side. Repeat. If all oil is absorbed, add a small amount and continue making crepes until no batter remains. If you have a bad sticking problem, use imitation grease.

Set crepes aside and keep warm.

Whip 1 cup heavy cream with 1 teaspoon sugar substitute and vanilla. Place whipped cream in center of crepe and roll crepe around it. Heat brandy in small

pan, ignite, and pour over crepes as you bring them
to the table.

Total Grams 34.5
Grams per serving 4.6

These crepes may also be served with preserves instead
of cream, or a combination of preserves mixed with
cream. Try them, too, with Zabaglione (see Index).

Chocolate Rum Charlotte

6 servings

1 envelope unflavored gelatin	sweetened chocolate
¾ cup cold water	¼ teaspoon salt
1¼ cups cream	1 teaspoon vanilla
1 tablespoon butter or margarine	1 teaspoon rum extract
1½ 1-ounce squares un-	1 teaspoon-equivalent sugar substitute

Soften gelatin in ¼ cup cold water.

Combine ¾ cup cream, ½ cup water, butter, and
chocolate in top of double boiler. Heat over simmering water.

Beat as it cooks with rotary beater until smooth and
well blended. Remove from heat. Blend in softened
gelatin, salt, vanilla, rum extract, and sugar substitute.
Blend well.

Chill until mixture is consistency of egg whites.

Whip ½ cup cream in small bowl until stiff. Fold
cream into chocolate gelatin mixture. Pour mixture
into mold. Chill until firm (about 2 hours).

For taste variation replace rum with 1 teaspoon vanilla.

Total Grams 22.7
Grams per serving 3.8

Zabaglione

6 servings

- 1 cup heavy cream
- 3 eggs, separated
- 1½ tablespoon-equivalents sugar substitute
- ¼ cup sherry
- 1 basket strawberries, washed and hulled

Scald heavy cream (do not boil). Beat egg yolks with 1 tablespoon sugar substitute. Pour cream over egg yolks and beat with wire whisk until well blended.

Cook mixture in top of double boiler, beating constantly with hand mixer or rotary beater until it begins to thicken. Cool.

Remove from heat and stir in sherry. Beat egg whites with remaining artificial sweetener until stiff. Fold into cream mixture carefully so that egg whites do not break down.

Refrigerate and serve with whole or sliced strawberries.

Total Grams 32.2
Grams per serving 5.5

A new version of a gourmet standard!

Dessert Fritters

2 servings

2 eggs, separated
1 teaspoon-equivalent brown sugar substitute
¾ teaspoon cinnamon
⅛ pound sweet butter, melted

Preheat oven to 350°.

Beat egg whites with sugar substitute until stiff. Add cinnamon to egg yolks, and fold into whites.

Melt butter in baking dish, and drop egg mixture by tablespoonfuls into it. Bake in 350° oven for 20 minutes. Cool.

2 tablespoons sweet butter
¼ teaspoon-equivalent brown sugar substitute
¼ teaspoon cinnamon
1 tablespoon brandy

Melt butter in skillet. Add sugar substitute and cinnamon. Fry fritters in butter until brown. Turn. Remove from heat.

Heat brandy in small pan. When hot, ignite, and pour over fritters. Serve at once.

Total Grams 7.5
Grams per serving 3.8

Great fun to serve!

Coconut Snowflakes

8 servings

1 recipe Vanilla Ice Cream (see Index)
2 tablespoons Cointreau
½ cup unsweetened coconut
1 tablespoon butter

Freeze ice cream in ice-cube trays with dividers left in.

Sprinkle Cointreau over coconut. Heat butter in skillet. Add coconut and sauté until light brown.

Remove firm ice cream from trays. Roll in coconut.

Top with Strawberry Sauce (see Index).

Total Grams   44.0
Grams per serving   5.5

Really cool!

Fruit Mold

8 servings

2 envelopes sugar-free raspberry gelatin
½ cup sliced strawberries
½ cup heavy cream, whipped

Prepare 1 package gelatin according to package directions. Add strawberries. Pour into mold. Chill until firm.

Prepare second package of gelatin without cold water. Cool. Fold in whipped cream.

Place on top of strawberry gelatin. Refrigerate for at least 2 hours.

To unmold: Run a wet knife along edge. Dip bottom of mold in warm water. Turn over onto wet plate.

Total Grams 17.0
Grams per serving 2.1

Lots more taste than carbohydrates!

Macadamia Nut Ice Cream

9 servings (½ cup each)

5 egg yolks
3 teaspoons vanilla
  extract
2½ tablespoons rum
2 tablespoon-
  equivalents sugar
  substitute

¼ cup water
½ cup coarsely chopped
  macadamia nuts
2 cups heavy cream,
  whipped

Place yolks, vanilla extract, rum, and sugar substitute, and water in blender.

Blend at medium speed for 30 seconds. Fold yolk mixture and chopped nuts into whipped cream.

Pour into refrigerator tray. Freeze for at least 4 hours.

Total Grams 59.4
Grams per serving 6.6

Delicious and crunchy!

Blueberry Ice Cream

9 servings (½ cup each)

5 egg yolks
3 teaspoons vanilla extract
2 tablespoon-equivalents white sugar substitute
¼ cup water
½ cup frozen blueberries, drained well
2 cups heavy cream, whipped

Place yolks, vanilla extract, sugar substitute, and water in blender. Blend at medium speed for 30 seconds. Add blueberries. Blend for 10 more seconds.

Fold yolk mixture into whipped cream. Blend lightly until you have marbled effect. Pour into freezer container. Freeze.

Total Grams 36.6
Grams per serving 4.0

So good—it'll chase all your blues away!

Vanilla Ice Cream

1 quart or 8 servings (½ cup each)

5 egg yolks
3 teaspoons vanilla extract
2 tablespoon-equivalents white sugar substitute
¼ cup water
2 cups heavy cream, whipped

Place yolks, vanilla extract, sugar substitute, and water in blender. Blend at medium speed for 30 seconds.

Fold yolk mixture into whipped cream. Be careful not to break down volume of whipped cream. Empty into refrigerator tray. Freeze for 2 hours.

> Total Grams 25.4
> Grams per serving 3.2

A very basic Dr. Atkins special!

Strawberry Ice Cream

10 servings

1 tablespoon fruit liqueur
4 tablespoon-equivalents sugar substitute
2 cups puréed strawberries
1½ cups heavy cream
2 inches vanilla bean, split and scraped
3 egg whites

Add liqueur and 2 tablespoons sugar substitute to strawberries Whip heavy cream with vanilla bean and 1 tablespoon sugar substitute. Fold strawberries into whipped cream, blending well. Separately beat egg whites until stiff with 1 tablespoon sugar substitute. Fold into cream mixture.

Spray ice cream mold with grease substitute.

Pour mixture into mold. Cover with transparent wrap and freeze for 2 hours. If in freezer for more than 6 hours before serving, allow to stand at room temperature for 15 minutes.

> Total Grams 55.9
> Grams per serving 5.6

Try it with Strawberry Sauce (see Index).

Blueberry-Raspberry Jam

12 tablespoons

1 tablespoon sugar-free raspberry gelatin
1 cup water
1 cup blueberries
1 teaspoon lemon juice
2 teaspoon-equivalents brown sugar substitute

Add gelatin to cold water. Bring to boil, stirring until completely dissolved.

Cool gelatin in refrigerator until it becomes consistency of egg whites. (This is done faster in freezer. If using this method, watch closely or it will become too thick.)

Heat blueberries in saucepan for about 5 minutes, or until tender. Remove from heat. Crush most of berries with fork. Leave some whole.

Stir for 2 minutes to cool.

Add lemon juice and brown sugar substitute to berries. Stir well. Fold berries into thickened gelatin. Mix well. Refrigerate until jellied.

Total Grams 36.8
Grams per tablespoon 3.1

Also great with Fluffy Jam Omelet (see Index)

Rhubarb-Strawberry Jelly

30 tablespoons

5 large stalks rhubarb
½ cup water
1 envelope sugar-free strawberry gelatin
1 cup fresh strawberries, halved and sliced

Cut off leaves and stem ends from rhubarb. Wash thoroughly. Dry well. If rhubarb is young, the skin is tender and will not need to be peeled. If skin is tough, peel rhubarb.

Cut rhubarb into ½-inch pieces. Place in large saucepan with water. Bring to boil. Lower heat and simmer, covered, for 15 minutes.

Stir in gelatin and strawberries.

Pour into jelly glasses and chill until set.

Total Grams   30.9
Grams per tablespoon   1.0

A tart-tasting treat!

Spicy Blueberry Jam

25 tablespoons

2 1-pint packages frozen blueberries
¼ cup wine vinegar
¼ teaspoon allspice
¼ teaspoon cloves
1 cinnamon stick
sugar substitute to taste

Put all ingredients except sugar substitute in heavy pan. Boil slowly for about ½ hour or until thick. Remove cloves and cinnamon stick. Store in refrigerator.

Total Grams   64.5
Grams per tablespoon   2.6

May be used as a topping for ice cream, custards, or as a filling for crepes or pancakes.

Blueberries with Heavy or Sour Cream

2 servings

½ cup blueberries, washed
4 teaspoon-equivalents brown sugar substitute
½ cup heavy cream

Mix blueberries with 1 tablespoon brown sugar substitute.

Whip heavy cream with 1 teaspoon brown sugar substitute. Fold blueberries and cream together. Serve.

Total Grams   16.4
Grams per serving   8.2

or

½ cup blueberries, washed
2 teaspoon-equivalents brown sugar substitute
½ cup sour cream

Follow above instructions.

Total Grams   17.7
Grams per serving   9.0

Have it "your way."

Strawberry Parfait

1 serving

2 scoops Ice Cream—Strawberry or Vanilla (see Index)
2 tablespoons Strawberry Sauce (see Index)

Alternate layers of ice cream with layers of strawberry sauce.

Top with fresh strawberry.

Total Grams   5.4

Really a favorite!

Lemon-Lime Mousse

8 servings

½ cup butter
9 egg yolks
 juice of 2 lemons
 juice of 2 limes
3 tablespoon-
 equivalents sugar
 substitute

2 teaspoons grated
 lemon rind
4 egg whites
1½ cups heavy cream
1 teaspoon vanilla
 extract

Melt butter in skillet.

Beat in egg yolks, one at a time, with wire whisk. Remove from heat. Add juice from lemons and limes, 2 tablespoons sugar substitute, and lemon rind. Beat well. Cool.

Beat egg whites with 2 teaspoons sugar substitute until stiff. Fold into lemon-lime mixture. Chill.

Whip heavy cream with 1 teaspoon sugar substitute and vanilla extract. Fold into chilled mixture. Refrigerate for at least 2 hours.

Total Grams 46.2
Grams per serving 5.8

Citrus flavor in a very special manner!

Butterscotch Cream Pudding

6 servings

1½ envelopes unflavored gelatin
6 ounces cold water
7 egg yolks, beaten
3 tablespoons butter
3 ounces cream
1½ teaspoons vanilla

3 tablespoon-equivalents brown sugar substitute
1½ teaspoon butterscotch extract
1½ cups heavy cream, whipped

Soften gelatin in 3 ounces water for 5 minutes.

Place yolks in double boiler. Add butter, cream, 3 ounces water, and gelatin. Do not allow water to boil; just simmer.

Stir constantly until mixture coats spoon. Cool.

Add vanilla, brown sugar substitute, and butterscotch extract. Fold in whipped cream.

Refrigerate before serving.

Total Grams 27.7
Grams per serving 4.6

Super flavor!

Chocolate Cream Debbie

10 servings

2 1-ounce squares un-
sweetened choco-
late, melted
2½ cups heavy cream
1 envelope unflavored
gelatin
¼ cup cold water
1 tablespoon crème de
cacao
2 tablespoon-

equivalents brown
sugar substitute
3 egg whites
2 inches vanilla bean,
split and scraped
1 tablespoon-
equivalent white
sugar substitute
1 Meringue Shell (see
Index) (optional)

Combine melted chocolate with 1 cup heavy cream.

Sprinkle gelatin over cold water. Add to chocolate
mixture and heat just to boiling. Allow to simmer for
about 2 minutes, stirring constantly. Do not boil.

Add crème de cacao and brown sugar substitute. Cool.
Beat egg whites until stiff. Fold into cooled chocolate
mixture. Pour into 10-inch pie plate. Refrigerate for
about ½ hour. Whip 1½ cups heavy cream with
vanilla bean and white sugar substitute. Top chocolate mixture with whipped cream. Refrigerate until
firm (about 2 hours).

Total Grams 39.6
Grams per serving 4.0

*Great when you want something sweet for late-night
snacks!*

Pumpkin Chiffon

8 servings

1 envelope unflavored
   gelatin
½ teaspoon salt
½ teaspoon nutmeg
½ teaspoon cinnamon
¼ teaspoon ginger
½ cup cold water
2 egg yolks, slightly
   beaten

1 cup heavy cream
1¼ cups canned pump-
   kin
2 tablespoon-
   equivalents brown
   sugar substitute
2 egg whites

Combine gelatin, salt, and spices. Add ¼ cup water. Stir. Mix egg yolks with heavy cream, ¼ cup water, and pumpkin in top of double boiler. Add gelatin mixture Cook over boiling water for 10 minutes, stirring constantly.

Refrigerate until thick as unbeaten egg whites. Stir occasionally. Add brown sugar substitute (taste for sweetness).

Beat egg whites until stiff. Fold chilled pumpkin mixture into egg whites. Be careful not to break down volume of egg whites. Turn into 1½ quart soufflé dish. Refrigerate.

Total Grams 30.2
Grams per serving 3.8

A light tasty delight!

Cheese Pudding

6 servings

2 eggs, slightly beaten
⅔ cup cream
½ cup grated Parmesan cheese
½ cup grated Swiss cheese
pinch each of salt and cayenne

Preheat oven to 450°.

Mix all ingredients together. Fill 6 small ramekins. Bake for 15 minutes in 450° oven.

Total Grams 10.9
Grams per serving 1.8

Keep it handy for easy snacks!

Coconut Drops

21 drops

1 cup shredded unsweetened coconut
1 tablespoon crème de cacao
3 egg whites, at room temperature
1 tablespoon-equivalent brown sugar substitute

Preheat oven to 400°.

Place coconut in bowl. Sprinkle crème de cacao over it and mix well.

In a separate bowl beat egg whites with brown sugar substitute until very stiff. Using a rubber scraper, fold whites into coconut with gentle under and over motion until all coconut is absorbed.

Drop by teaspoonfuls onto cookie sheet that has been sprayed with grease substitute.

Bake in 400° oven for 7 to 10 minutes. Cool. Refrigerate to store.

Total Grams 25.9
Grams per serving 1.0

(Unsweetened coconut may be purchased in health-food stores or you may buy a fresh coconut, crack it open, and shred the meat.)

The "Pop" Pop

6 Popsicles

1½ cups sugar-free fruit-flavored soda
6 teaspoons cream
sprinkle of sugar substitute (optional)

Mix all ingredients together.

Fill plastic molds for Popsicles (1 mold holds 6 Popsicles) with mixture. Insert stick if desired. (It is best to do this when Popsicles are partially frozen.)

Freeze.

Total Grams 2.6
Grams per serving .4

The art of delicious "Pops."

Pink Lady

4 servings

1 package unflavored gelatin
4 tablespoons cold water
8 ounces sugar-free strawberry soda
1 cup heavy cream
1 tablespoon-equivalent sugar substitute

Sprinkle gelatin onto cold water. When it begins to thicken, add to strawberry soda.

Heat this mixture in top of double boiler until gelatin dissolves, stirring constantly.

Refrigerate until mixture begins to thicken.

Whip heavy cream until stiff with sugar substitute.

Fold gelatin mixture into whipped cream and refrigerate until firm.

Total Grams 8.2
Grams per serving 2.1

Great if you've got the diet blues.

Coconut Drops Bernier

10 candies

1 recipe Coconut Drops (see Index)
½ recipe Spicy Blueberry Jam (see Index)
1 tablespoon kirsch liqueur
2 egg yolks, beaten
hot oil

Press in bottom of coconut drops and fill cavity with jam. Sandwich together in pairs. Sprinkle with a few drops of kirsch.

Dip each pair into egg yolks and fry in deep fat (370°) until lightly browned. Drain on absorbent paper. Serve hot.

Total Grams 43.6
Grams per serving 4.0

A really unusual treat!

Peanut Butter Cookies

40 cookies

½ cup chunk-style peanut butter
¾ cup cream
½ cup chopped pecans
2 teaspoons vanilla
2 teaspoon-equivalents
sugar substitute

2 tablespoons soya
powder
1 teaspoon baking powder

Preheat oven to 375°.

Spray a cookie sheet with grease substitute.

Mix all ingredients in bowl. Blend well.

Drop on cookie sheet by teaspoonfuls. Bake for about 10 minutes.

Total Grams 52.7
Grams per cookie 1.3

Keep the cookie jar full!

Peanut Butter Dreams

36 balls

1 egg, well beaten
⅓ cup chunk-style peanut butter
1 tablespoon soft sweet butter
1 teaspoon vanilla
1 tablespoon-equivalent brown sugar substitute
¾ cup finely chopped walnuts

Mix all ingredients except nuts together well. Shape into small balls. Roll balls in chopped nuts.

Refrigerate until firm.

Total Grams 46.2
Grams per ball 1.3

A flavor treat for grown-up kids!

Chocolate Fudge

15 squares

1 package diet chocolate pudding (without sugar)
2 tablespoon-equivalents brown sugar substitute
½ cup heavy cream
1 tablespoon crème de cacao
3 heaping tablespoons chunk-style peanut butter

Mix all ingredients together except peanut butter. Place over low flame and add peanut butter. Heat until peanut butter melts. Stir until well blended.

Grease spray a small baking pan. Spoon mixture into pan.

Refrigerate until firm. Slice into at least 15 squares.

Total Grams 28.3
Grams per square 1.9

Oh, fudge—I love it!

Chocolate Almonds

6 candies

2 1-ounce squares unsweetened chocolate
2 tablespoons crème de cacao
2 tablespoons water
1 tablespoon-equivalent brown sugar substitute
2 tablespoons salted almonds with skins

Melt chocolate over water in double boiler. Stir. Add crème de cacao and water and stir well. Add brown sugar substitute. Stir. Add almonds and stir well.

Drop by teaspoonfuls onto cookie sheet that has been sprayed with grease substitute. Refrigerate.

Total Grams 29.1
Grams per serving 5.0

A sweet-tooth satisfier!

Deep Fried Camembert and Cantaloupe

6 servings

1 small cantaloupe or casaba, peeled, seeded, and cut
into large cubes
1 Camembert cheese, cut into 12 pieces
3 eggs, beaten
1 bag fried pork rinds, crushed
oil (for deep fat)

Dip cantaloupe and cheese into eggs and then into pork rinds.

Deep fry in very hot oil for 30 seconds.

Total Grams 38.2
Grams per serving 6.4

A taste surprise!

Brownies

30 squares

½ cup butter, at room
temperature
2 eggs
2 1-ounce squares un-
sweetened chocolate
2 teaspoons chocolate
extract
2 tablespoons water
2 tablespoons soya
powder

½ cup coarsely chopped
walnuts
2 tablespoon-equivalents
brown sugar sub-
stitute
3 tablespoons crème
de cacao

Preheat oven to 350°.

Cream butter with electric hand mixer. Add eggs one at a time, beating well.

Melt chocolate with extract and water in top of double boiler. (If it gets too thick, add a little more water.) Add melted chocolate, soya powder, chopped walnuts, and brown sugar substitute to butter. Mix well.

Grease a 1½-quart flat baking dish.

Pour in chocolate mixture. Bake in 350° oven for 15 minutes. Do not overcook. Remove from oven.

Sprinkle crème de cacao over top. Cool. Cut into at least 30 squares.

Total Grams 59.9
Grams per square 2.0

An old favorite.

Cottage Cheese Custard

6 servings

⅔ cup water
1⅓ cups cream
1 cup cottage cheese
3 eggs
¼ teaspoon salt
sugar substitute

1 teaspoon grated lemon rind
1 tablespoon crème de cacao
cinnamon (optional)

Preheat oven to 300°.

Mix water and cream in saucepan; scald, but do not allow to boil.

Place cottage cheese, eggs, salt, lemon rind, and crème de cacao in blender.

Blend for 1 minute at high speed. Add ½ cream mixture. Blend. Add remaining cream mixture, and blend well at high speed.

Fill 6 buttered custard cups with custard and place in shallow pan half filled with warm water. Sprinkle with cinnamon and sugar substitute. Bake in 300° oven for 40 minutes or until custard is set and lightly browned.

Total Grams 28.8
Grams per serving 4.8

Pretty Ginger Ale Mold

6 servings

1 envelope sugar-free lemon-flavored gelatin
2 cups sugar-free ginger ale
1 cup cantaloupe balls
¼ cup chopped walnuts

Dissolve gelatin in ½ cup ginger ale. Bring to boil. Stir. Be sure gelatin completely dissolves. Cool.

Add remaining 1½ cups ginger ale. Chill until consistency of egg whites.

Fold in cantaloupe balls and walnuts. Pour into wet mold. Chill.

Total Grams 27.2
Grams per serving 4.5

Really worth the trouble!

Mock Choc Coffee Cream

6 servings

3 cups ricotta cheese
1 tablespoon instant coffee
1 tablespoon cognac or brandy
2 tablespoon-equivalents sugar substitute
4 tablespoons heavy cream
vanilla

Combine all ingredients. Beat until smooth.

Chill for 1 hour. Serve.

Total Grams 43.2
Grams per serving 7.2

Nothing mock about the flavor!

BEVERAGES

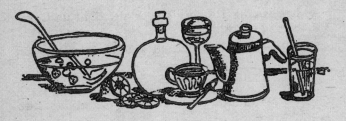

Instant Iced Coffee

1 serving

3 ice cubes
4 tablespoons cream
⅛ teaspoon-equivalent sugar substitute
½ cup water
½ teaspoon powdered coffee

Place all ingredients in blender at high speed for 30 to 40 seconds.

Total Grams 1.8

Refreshing on a hot summer day!

Cappuccino

1 serving

1 recipe Hot Chocolate (see next page)
½ teaspoon instant coffee
½ teaspoon brandy extract
1 cinnamon stick

Make hot chocolate. Add coffee and brandy extract.

Serve in mug with cinnamon stick.

Total Grams 5.1

Serve it when company comes!

Hot Chocolate

1 serving

⅓ cup cream
⅔ cup water
1 teaspoon unsweetened cocoa
1 teaspoon-equivalent sugar substitute
½ teaspoon vanilla

Place all ingredients in saucepan. Heat to boiling point, but do not boil. Stir constantly.

Serve in mug.

Total Grams 5.1

For chilly wintry nights!

Spicy Cocktail

2 servings

2 cups beef broth
4 teaspoons tomato sauce
½ teaspoon onion juice or grated onion
½ teaspoon Worcestershire sauce
1 or two drops Tabasco sauce

Combine all ingredients. Mix well. Serve hot or cold.

Total Grams 3.0
Grams per person 1.5

Orange Cooler

4 servings

1 package sugar-free orange gelatin	1 teaspoon orange extract
2 egg whites, beaten stiff	2 tablespoon-equivalents sugar substitute
2 teaspoons grated lemon rind	4 strawberries
	4 ice cubes

4 lemon slices

Prepare gelatin according to package directions and cool.

Beat in stiff egg whites with wire whisk.

Add lemon rind, orange extract, and sugar substitute. Place in blender. Add strawberries and ice cubes. Blend at medium speed for 30 seconds.

Pour into glasses and garnish with lemon slices.

Total Grams 10.2
Grams per serving 2.5

Delicious for breakfast!

Ice Cream Soda

1 serving

⅔ glass any diet soda
2 scoops Vanilla Ice Cream (see Index)

Total Grams 4.7

Blender-Thick Raspberry Shake

2 servings

2 scoops Vanilla Ice Cream (see Index)
3 tablespoons heavy cream
2 tablespoons sugar-free diet raspberry syrup*
1 8-ounce bottle sugar-free ginger ale

Place ingredients in blender. Blend for 1 minute at medium speed.

Total Grams   7.9
Grams per serving   4.0

* We have used No-Cal syrups.

It's the raspberries!

Chocolate Shake

1 serving

1 envelope unflavored
  gelatin
1 cup sugar-free
  chocolate soda
1 tablespoon
  unsweetened cocoa

4 ice cubes
1/3 cup heavy cream
1 teaspoon-equivalent
  sugar substitute
- dash of salt

Place gelatin, 1/4 cup soda, and cocoa in saucepan. Stir well.

Heat slowly to boiling point. Be sure gelatin dissolves completely. Cool.

Place ice cubes in blender. Add cooled gelatin mixture, heavy cream, 3/4 cup soda, sugar substitute, and salt.

Blend at high speed for 30 seconds.

Serve in tall glass. It will become thicker as it sets. Stir vigorously.

Total Grams 6.1

Sweet-tooth satisfying!

Shape-Up Shake

1 serving

- 1 envelope sugar-free lime gelatin
- 1 cup sugar-free diet soda
- 4 ice cubes
- ⅓ cup heavy cream
- 1 teaspoon-equivalent sugar substitute

Place gelatin and ¼ cup soda in saucepan. Heat to boiling point, stirring constantly. Be sure gelatin dissolves. Cool.

Place ice cubes in blender, add gelatin mixture, heavy cream, ¾ cup soda, and sugar substitute.

Blend at high speed for 30 seconds.

Serve in tall glass. It will become thicker as it sets. Stir vigorously.

Total Grams 3.0

LOW FAT RECIPES

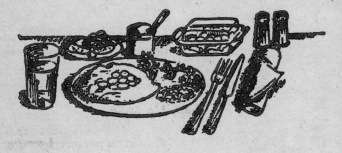

Spicy Mushroom Appetizer

6 servings

1 pound large mushrooms	½ cup safflower oil
½ onion, minced	¼ cup tarragon vinegar
2 tablespoons minced chives	¼ cup Sauterne
¼ teaspoon minced tarragon	½ large clove garlic
	1 teaspoon lemon juice

Wash and trim mushrooms. Dry well and slice thin.

Combine remaining ingredients and pour over mushrooms.

Marinate in refrigerator for at least 1 hour or keep them for days to snack on.

Total Grams 33.6
Grams per serving 5.6

Great on salads or cold meat.

Cottage Cheese Omelet

1 serving

¼ cup egg substitute*
¼ cup cottage cheese
¼ teaspoon seasoned salt
½ teaspoon caraway seeds
1 teaspoon corn oil margarine
2 egg whites, beaten stiff

Mix together egg substitute, cottage cheese, salt, and caraway seeds.

Melt margarine in skillet. Fold cottage cheese mixture into stiff egg whites and place in skillet.

Allow to set. Stir with fork, and repeat until desired doneness.

Total Grams 2.6

• We have used Fleischmann's Egg Beaters.

Eggplant Omelet

4 servings

  1 cup diced eggplant
  4 tablespoons corn oil margarine
  ¼ teaspoon garlic powder
  ½ cup tomato sauce
  1½ cups egg substitute
  ½ teaspoon seasoned salt

Peel eggplant. Cut into small cubes and soak in bowl of cold water for ½ hour. Dry eggplant well.

Melt 3 tablespoons margarine in skillet. Add eggplant and garlic powder. Sauté until eggplant begins to brown. Add tomato sauce. Set aside.

Place 1 tablespoon margarine in large skillet and allow to melt over very low heat. Add egg substitute and continue to cook over low heat until they set.

Spoon eggplant mixture onto egg substitute and either fold it over or roll it up.

Total Grams 18.7
Grams per serving 4.7

Spanish Omelet

1 serving

½ cup egg substitute
1 tablespoon corn oil
   margarine
1 tablespoon chopped
   onion
½ teaspoon seasoned salt

1 tablespoon chopped
   green pepper
2 tablespoons diced
   tomato
dash of chili powder
   (optional)

Prepare egg substitute for scrambled eggs.

Melt margarine in skillet. Sauté onion, salt, pepper, tomato, and chili powder for 2 minutes. Add egg substitute.

Allow to set. Stir with fork, and repeat until desired doneness.

Total Grams 6.0

Peppers and Eggs

1 serving

1 green pepper
1 tablespoon oil
⅛ teaspoon onion powder
½ cup egg substitute

Cut pepper in half lengthwise and remove seeds. Cut into 6 pieces lengthwise.

Heat oil in small skillet. Add peppers. Sauté until soft. Add onion powder and egg substitute. Allow eggs to set for 1 minute. Stir. Allow eggs to set again, and stir as you would scrambled eggs. Repeat until desired consistency.

Total Grams   7.2

Quick and delicious for breakfast or a late supper.

Tasty Tender Flank Steak

4 servings

1 clove garlic, minced	¼ teaspoon pepper
1 cup vegetable oil	2 teaspoons dry mustard
½ cup vinegar	2 teaspoons Worcester-
1 teaspoon salt	shire sauce

1 flank steak, scored

Combine all ingredients except steak. Place steak in sauce. Set for 4 hours in shallow covered pan. Remove steak and broil for 4 minutes on each side. Carve diagonally across grain in thin slices.

Total Grams   7.2
Grams per serving   1.8

This is a delicious budget dish.

Super Steak

6 servings

3 cloves garlic, minced
2 tablespoons safflower oil
2 tablespoons wine vinegar
¼ cup dry red wine
½ teaspoon seasoned salt
3 pounds lean steak

Combine garlic, oil, vinegar, wine, and salt in shallow dish large enough to hold meat.

Add meat and allow to marinate for at least 2 hours. Turn often.

Remove steak from marinade and broil to desired doneness.

	Total Grams	Trace
	Grams per serving	Trace

Cool Finland Veal

6 servings

3 pounds veal (shoulder, breast, or neck)	2 tablespoons vinegar
	2 bay leaves
4 tablespoons chopped onion	4 teaspoons salt
	boiling water
8 whole allspice	½ teaspoon parsley

Cut meat into 3-inch cubes. Add some bone.

In large pot place veal, onion, allspice, vinegar, bay leaves, and salt. Add boiling water to cover. Remove any foam that comes to the top as it is cooking. Simmer until tender, for about 1½ hours. Allow meat to cook in broth.

Remove meat from bones, and cut into ½-inch pieces. Set aside. Strain broth.

Pour ½ broth into 1½- to 2-quart mold. Chill mold until broth is the consistency of egg whites. Add diced meat and remaining broth. Return to refrigerator until set (for about 24 hours). Unmold on platter. Garnish with parsley.

Total Grams   6.2
Grams per serving   1.0

Veal with Tuna Sauce (Vitello Tonnato)

6 servings

3 pounds boneless leg of veal in 1 piece
1 13-ounce can tuna fish
2 tablespoons diced onion
10 anchovy fillets, chopped

1 cup dry white wine
1 cup chicken broth
4 tablespoons safflower oil
2 teaspoons tarragon vinegar

salt and pepper to taste

Tie meat with string to hold together.

Place veal, tuna fish, onion, anchovies, wine, and chicken broth in large pot. Cover and simmer over low heat for about 2½ hours.

Remove meat and place in bowl. Put gravy from pot in blender. Add oil, vinegar, salt, and pepper. Blend at low speed for 30 seconds.

Pour marinade over meat, cover, and refrigerate for 2 days.

Slice meat thin, and serve at room temperature with a little of the marinade.

Total Grams   7.9
Grams per serving   1.3

Delicate Italian flavoring!

Lamb Patties in Tomato Sauce

4 servings

2 pounds very lean
  ground lamb
½ cup egg substitute
2 cloves garlic
¼ teaspoon cinnamon
1 teaspoon cumin

1½ teaspoons salt
½ teaspoon pepper
2 tablespoons corn or
  safflower oil
1 8-ounce can tomato
  sauce

1 can water

Combine first 7 ingredients to make patties, but use
½ teaspoon cumin.

In large skillet sauté patties on both sides in hot oil.
Remove from skillet.

Pour tomato sauce, water, and ½ teaspoon cumin into
skillet. Simmer for 10 minutes.

Return lamb to skillet and simmer, covered, for 10
more minutes.

Total Grams 14.8
Grams per serving 3.7

Roman Egg Beaters

4 servings

1 tablespoon corn or
  safflower oil
½ cup raw lean ground
  beef
1 cup chopped fresh
  spinach
1 clove garlic, minced
1½ cups egg substitute

3 tablespoons white
  wine
2 tablespoons grated
  Parmesan cheese
1 teaspoon basil
  salt and pepper to
  taste

Heat oil in skillet and sauté ground beef, breaking in smaller pieces as it cooks. As it starts to brown add spinach and garlic. Cover for 4 or 5 minutes.

Place egg substitute in bowl, and add wine, cheese, basil, salt, and pepper. Mix well.

Cooking at the lowest heat, pour egg substitute mixture over ground beef mixture. Mix well, allowing egg substitute to set firmly.

If ground beef is too oily after sautéing, pour off extra fat.

Total Grams 14.3
Grams per serving 3.6

Salmon à la Napolitana

4 servings

6 salmon fillets	⅔ can water
4 tablespoons olive oil	¼ teaspoon basil
1 small onion	½ teaspoon oregano
1 8-ounce can tomato sauce	¼ teaspoon-equivalent sugar substitute

Preheat oven to 350°.

Sauté salmon fillets in 2 tablespoons olive oil. Place in baking dish.

Sauté onion in 2 tablespoons olive oil. When light brown, add tomato sauce and water. Cook for 15 minutes.

Add basil, oregano, and sugar substitute, and cook for 5 more minutes.

Pour onion mixture over salmon.

Bake in 350° oven for 20 minutes.

Total Grams   18.1
Grams per serving   4.5

A real quicky!

Oven-Barbecued Chicken

6 servings

1 3-pound chicken, cut up	½ teaspoon paprika
1 teaspoon seasoned salt	2 tablespoons lime juice
¼ teaspoon Tabasco sauce	2 tablespoons safflower oil
1 teaspoon dried tarragon	

Preheat oven to 350°.

Prepare chicken by washing and drying well.

Mix salt, Tabasco sauce, paprika, lime juice, oil, and tarragon together. Place chicken in baking dish. Pour oil mixture over chicken.

Marinate in refrigerator for 2 hours. Return to room temperature. Bake in 350° oven for 1 hour. Turn once. Baste every 10 minutes.

Total Grams   2.2
Grams per serving   .4

Very crispy and good!

Chicken and Tuna

2 servings

4 chicken cutlets, boned
  and skin removed
½ teaspoon seasoned salt
2 tablespoons corn oil
  margarine
4 heaping tablespoons
  flaked tuna fish

4 tablespoons dry white
  wine
½ teaspoon dried tarragon
8 thin slices skim milk
  mozzarella cheese

Wash chicken and pat dry. Sprinkle with salt.

Melt margarine in skillet and sauté chicken to desired doneness. Remove to broiler pan.

Mix tuna, wine, and tarragon together. Spoon onto cooked chicken. Top with mozzarella slices and place under broiler until cheese melts.

Total Grams 7.0
Grams per serving 3.5

West Indian Chicken Creole

4 servings

1 2½-pound broiler-fryer,
  cut up and skin
  removed
2 tablespoons lemon
  juice
½ teaspoon pepper
½ teaspoon seasoned salt
2 tablespoons low fat
  soya powder

3 tablespoons corn oil
  margarine
1 large onion, sliced
1 cup chicken broth
1 large tomato, cut into
  chunks

Wash and dry chicken.

Combine lemon juice, pepper, salt, and soya powder. Roll chicken in mixture until well coated.

Melt margarine in large skillet and sauté onion and chicken until well browned on all sides. Add broth and tomato. Simmer, covered, over low heat for 1 hour. Stir often.

Total Grams 31.2
Grams per serving 8.0

Baked Tomato

1 serving

1 small tomato
½ tablespoon corn oil margarine
    onion salt

Preheat oven to 350°.

Make a slit in top of tomato and insert margarine. Sprinkle well with onion salt. Bake in small dish with small amount of water in the bottom for 15 minutes.

Total Grams 6.0

Green Bean Quiche

8 servings

3 tablespoons corn or safflower oil
½ cup onion
½ cup mushrooms
1 pound very lean ground beef
1 pound fresh green beans, cooked and drained

1½ teaspoons salt
½ teaspoon pepper
½ teaspoon nutmeg
1½ cups egg substitute
1 tablespoon lemon juice
⅛ teaspoon sugar substitute

Preheat oven to 325°.

In a skillet heat oil. Sauté onion for 3 minutes in oil, and add mushrooms. Stir until lightly browned.

Add meat to skillet. Break up slowly until browned.

Add green beans, salt, pepper, and nutmeg. Stir. Cool for 10 minutes.

Mix egg substitute, lemon juice, and sugar substitute together in a bowl. Add to meat mixture.

Oil a pie plate and fill with meat mixture. Bake in 325° oven for 45 minutes until browned and set.

Serve hot or cold.

Total Grams 43.9
Grams per serving 5.5

Quick Italian Supper

3 servings

2 tablespoons safflower oil	1 teaspoon basil
2 stalks celery, diced	1 cup egg substitute
1 zucchini, diced	2 tablespoons grated
1 small clove garlic, minced	Parmesan cheese
1 tomato, skinned and diced	salt and pepper to taste

Heat oil in skillet, and brown celery and zucchini well.

Add garlic in last 2 minutes.

Add tomato, and simmer for 15 minutes, adding basil for last 5 minutes.

Add egg substitute, Parmesan cheese, salt, and pepper. Cover skillet, and cook slowly for about 10 minutes.

Turn over for a few minutes to brown other side lightly.

Total Grams 22.1
Grams per serving 7.4

It's a matter of timing.

Leftover Veal Salad

6 servings

2 cups diced cold roast
veal
1½ cups diced celery
4 tablespoons chopped
scallions
1½ teaspoons dried
tarragon

¾ cup shredded green
pepper
¾ cup sliced fresh
mushrooms
1 cup safflower oil
mayonnaise
lettuce leaves

Combine first 7 ingredients. Mix very well.

Serve on lettuce leaves.

Total Grams 28.5
Grams per serving 4.7

Good to the last drop!

Tuna and Eggs

2 servings

1 6½-ounce can tuna fish
1 cup egg substitute
dash of garlic salt
1 teaspoon chopped
parsley

3 anchovy fillets, minced
salt and pepper to taste
2 tablespoons oil

Place tuna fish in bowl and break into small pieces.

Add egg substitute, garlic salt, parsley, anchovy fillets, salt, and pepper. Mix well.

In skillet heat oil, add egg mixture, and simmer on low heat, covered, for about 10 minutes. Turn and brown lightly on other side for a few minutes.

If you have trouble turning omelette, cut in half and turn ½ at a time.

Serve.

Total Grams 3.6
Grams per serving 1.8

Green Peppers and Mushrooms

8 servings

3 tablespoons corn or safflower oil
½ cup thinly sliced onion
1 clove garlic, minced
1 pound green peppers
½ pound mushrooms, sliced

3 tablespoons tomato sauce
½ teaspoon oregano
1 teaspoon salt
dash of pepper

Heat oil in skillet. Sauté onion for 5 minutes. Add garlic and peppers, stirring frequently for about 10 minutes.

Add mushrooms and stir until lightly browned, for about 10 minutes.

Add tomato sauce, oregano, salt, and pepper.

Simmer over low heat for about 5 minutes, stirring frequently.

Total Grams   49.7
Grams per serving   6.3

Delicious used in an omelet or over hamburgers.

Tomato Aspic with Tuna

2 servings

1 teaspoon unflavored gelatin
½ cup cold water
½ cup tomato juice
½ teaspoon Worcestershire sauce
2 tablespoons tarragon vinegar
dash of paprika

¼ teaspoon seasoned salt
1 teaspoon onion juice
1 teaspoon lemon juice
½ cup flaked tuna fish (water packed)
1 tablespoon diced celery
1 tablespoon diced green pepper
2 lettuce leaves

Sprinkle gelatin over cold water.

Heat tomato juice to boil and pour into gelatin. Add Worcestershire sauce, vinegar, paprika, salt, onion juice, and lemon juice. Cool until the consistency of egg whites.

Add tuna, celery, and green pepper.

Fill mold. Chill until firm. Serve on lettuce leaves.

Total Grams   10.2
Grams per serving   5.1

Cottage Caesar

4 servings

1 recipe Dressing of the House, made with safflower oil
   (see Index)
1 quart romaine lettuce leaves, washed and dried
½ cup chopped celery
½ cup thinly sliced cucumber
1 cup coarsely chopped fried pork rinds
1 pound creamed cottage cheese (2 cups)

Place dressing in bottom of large salad bowl.

Rip lettuce into bite-size pieces. Add to salad bowl.
Add celery, cucumber, and pork rinds. Toss well.

Divide into individual servings. Top with scoop of
cottage cheese.

Total Grams   34.2
Grams per serving   8.5

Caesar never had it so good!

Island Cottage Cheese

2 servings

½ pound cottage cheese (1 cup)
½ cup sliced strawberries
¼ teaspoon mint leaves
   sugar substitute to taste
2 tablespoons unsweetened coconut

Combine cottage cheese, strawberries, mint leaves, and
sugar substitute.

Top with coconut.

Total Grams 14.2
Grams per serving 7.0

Really something else!

Blender Dressing for Greens

2½ cups

1 clove garlic, peeled
1 stalk celery, chopped
½ medium onion, sliced
1 2-ounce can flat
   anchovies
1 teaspoon seasoned salt
10 turns of pepper mill
¼ teaspoon sugar
   substitute

2 tablespoons Dijon
   mustard
juice of half a lemon
   (about 1 tablespoon)
2 cups polyunsaturated
   oil
½ cup egg substitute

Put garlic, celery, onion, anchovies, salt, pepper, sugar substitute, mustard, and lemon in blender. Purée.

Add oil to dressing and blend until smooth. Add egg substitute and blend a few seconds longer.

Total Grams 13.2

Blueberry Whip

6 servings

1 cup fresh or frozen unsweetened blueberries
4 teaspoon-equivalents sugar substitute
2 egg whites
⅛ teaspoon salt

Mash blueberries slightly with 1 tablespoon sugar substitute.

Beat egg whites with salt and 1 teaspoon sugar substitute. Allow them to get stiff, but not dry.

Fold berries into egg whites; pile into compote dishes. Serve immediately.

Total Grams 36.8
Grams per serving 6.1

Takes no time at all!

Cottage Cheese and Fruit

2 servings

2 scoops cottage cheese (½ cup)
½ cup honeydew melon balls
¼ cup raspberries
4 tablespoons Poppy Seed Dessert Dressing, made with safflower oil (see Index)

Place scoop of cottage cheese in middle of plate. Top with melon balls and raspberries. Pour on dessert dressing.

Total Grams 14.5
Grams per serving 7.3

A cool and refreshing dessert!

Coffee Foam

6 servings

2 envelopes unflavored gelatin
2 cups strong hot coffee
8 teaspoon-equivalents brown sugar substitute
3 egg whites, at room temperature

Place gelatin, coffee, and 6 teaspoons brown sugar substitute in blender. Blend at low speed until gelatin dissolves. Pour into dish and refrigerate until *slightly* thickened. Beat egg whites until stiff with remaining 2 teaspoons brown sugar substitute.

Fold coffee mixture into egg whites. Refrigerate.

Total Grams 3.2
Grams per serving .5

A first week treat!

Cantaloupe and Wine

8 servings

2 small cantaloupes
1 envelope sugar-free lime gelatin
1 cup boiling water
2 teaspoon-equivalents sugar substitute
1 cup cold dry white wine

Cut cantaloupes in half and scoop out seeds. Refrigerate.

Add gelatin to water and stir until completely dissolved. Take off fire. Add sugar substitute and cold wine to gelatin. Mix well.

Refrigerate until gelatin is a heavy syrup.

Spoon into cantaloupe halves and allow to set in refrigerator. Cut into quarters and serve.

Total Grams   47.8
Grams per serving   6.0

Different and delicious!

Strawberry Ambrosia

6 servings

½ cup unsweetened coconut
1 tablespoon Cointreau
1 basket strawberries, washed and hulled
2 teaspoon-equivalents sugar substitute

Place coconut in bowl. Sprinkle with Cointreau. Mix well. Sprinkle strawberries with sugar substitute. Place in serving dishes and top with coconut.

Total Grams   34.5
Grams per serving   5.8

Red, white, and perfect!

Glazed Strawberries

6 servings

2 tablespoons sugar-free diet raspberry syrup
2 tablespoons kirschwasser liqueur
2 cups whole strawberries

Heat syrup and liqueur just to boiling.

Pour over strawberries, toss gently, and serve.

Total Grams 39.0
Grams per serving 6.5

Something extra special with no special effort!

Strawberry Sponge

4 servings

1 envelope sugar-free strawberry gelatin
¼ cup cold water
½ cup hot water
½ cup sugar-free strawberry soda

1½ tablespoons lemon juice
2 egg whites, beaten stiff
1 teaspoon-equivalent sugar substitute
mint sprigs

Sprinkle gelatin over cold water. Add hot water and stir until gelatin dissolves. Add soda and lemon juice. Refrigerate until it begins to thicken. Beat with electric hand mixer until frothy.

Beat egg whites with sugar substitute and fold into gelatin mixture.

Serve in parfait glasses. Garnish with mint sprigs.

Total Grams 4.0
Grams per serving 1.0

Filled with flavor!

Meringue Munchies

10 munchies

2 egg whites
¼ teaspoon seasoned salt
¼ cup pecans (crushed in blender)

Preheat oven to 250°.

Beat egg whites with salt until *very* stiff.

Fold in pecans. Be very careful not to break down stiff egg whites.

Grease cookie sheet. Drop egg white mixture by table-spoonfuls onto cookie sheet.

Bake in 250° oven for 1 hour. Turn off oven and allow to sit for ½ hour.

Total Grams 4.0
Grams per serving .4

Use in place of crackers or as snack.

Strawberry-Lemon Meringue Pie

10 servings

4 cups whole strawberries
   (about 2 cups mea-
   sured after puréed)
3 egg yolks
1 cup boiling water
1 envelope diet strawberry
   gelatin
1 teaspoon strawberry
   extract

1 teaspoon grated lemon
   peel
7 egg whites, beaten stiff
2 tablespoon-equivalents
   white sugar substitute
1 Meringue Shell (see
   Index) (optional)

Preheat oven to 450°.

Place strawberries and egg yolks in blender and purée. Boil water and add gelatin. Stir until dissolved. Add extract, lemon peel, and strawberries. Cook for about 2 minutes, stirring constantly. Cool.

Beat egg whites with sugar substitute until stiff. Fold half of egg whites into strawberry mixture. Pour mixture into round cake pan. Top with remaining egg whites. Be careful to cover strawberry mixture completely and seal around edges. Cook for 7 to 10 minutes in 450° oven or until brown.

Allow pie to cool before you refrigerate. Refrigerate at least 2 hours before serving.

(A few drops of red food coloring will give strawberry mixture a deeper color if desired.)

Total Grams   45.0
Grams per serving   4.5

Really delightful!

Meringue Shell

6 meringues

     4 egg whites
     pinch of salt
     4 teaspoons crème de cacao

Preheat oven to 250°.

Place egg whites and salt in bowl. Beat together until frothy. Gradually add crème de cacao. Continue beating until whites are stiff, glossy, and stand in stiff peaks.

Grease 6 muffin tins. Fill cups with meringue, hollowing out top with back of spoon.

Bake in 250° oven for 1 hour.

The How-tos of Beating Eggs for Meringues:

The amount can be varied in this recipe. Allow 1 egg white to 1 teaspoon crème de cacao. Eggs will beat better at room temperature, but separate better when cold. The trick is to separate them when cold, then let stand until they reach room temperature.

The best way to beat eggs is with a hand electric beater; however, a rotary beater will also do the job.

Total Grams   16.0
Grams per meringue   3.0

It's all in knowing how to!

RESTAURANT MENUS

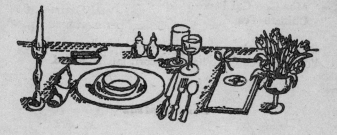

Suggested Dinners from Chinese Menu

Seafood Balls
Chicken in Foil
Har Kew
Chinese Tea

Stuffed Shrimp
Barbecued Spareribs
Chicken Soup with Chinese Vegetables
Moo Goo Gai Pan
Chinese Tea

Oriental foods are offered in large variety on this diet.
You must be sure to have the cornstarch omitted.

Chinese Menu

Appetizers
Seafood Shrimp
Stuffed Shrimp
Chicken in Foil
Barbecued Chicken Wings
Barbecued Spareribs
Barbecued Pork

Soups
Egg Drop Soup (without cornstarch)
Clear Chicken Broth
Chicken Soup with Chinese Vegetables
Chinese Mustard Greens with Ham

MAIN DISHES

Seafood
Shrimp, Lobster, or Crabmeat Ding
Lobster Cantonese
Shrimp with Lobster Sauce

Lobster Kew
Shrimp with Tomatoes and Peppers
Shrimp with Bean Sprouts
Seafood Go Ba (without rice)
Har Kew
Lobster or Crabmeat Soong (pass on rice noodles)

Poultry
Chicken Curry
Chicken with Tomatoes and Peppers
Chicken with Oyster Sauce
Pressed Duck and Mushroom Sauce
Chicken Kew
Moo Goo Gai Pan
Almond Dice Cut Chicken

Pork
Roast Pork with Mixed Chinese Vegetables
Almond Roast Pork Ding
Roast Pork with Bean Sprouts
Roast Pork with Mushrooms
Roast Pork with Snow Pea Pods
Roast Pork with Pepper and Tomatoes

Beef
Pepper Steak
Pepper Steak with Tomatoes
Beef with Bean Sprouts
Beef with Mixed Chinese Vegetables
Beef with Oyster Sauce
Beef Curry
Beef with Snow Pea Pods
Beef Soong
Steak Kew
Kowloon Steak

Egg Foo Yung
Roast Pork Egg Foo Yung
Chicken Egg Foo Yung
Shrimp Egg Foo Yung

Lobster Egg Foo Yung
Egg Foo Yung Cantonese
Subgum Egg Foo Yung
Vegetable Egg Foo Yung
Ham Egg Foo Yung
Crabmeat Egg Foo Yung

Vegetables
Sautéed Snow Pea Pods
Sautéed Mixed Chinese Vegetables
Sautéed Bean Sprouts

Beverage
Chinese Tea

Suggested Dinners from French Menu

Bouillabaisse
Veal Cordon-Bleu
Épinard à la Crème
Mixed Green Salad
Cheese
Demitasse

Pâté Maison
Soupe à l'Oignon
Chateaubriand Bordelaise
Ratatouille
Strawberries and Cream
Coffee

French Menu

Appetizers
Pâté Maison
Avocado Vinaigrette
Clams Mignonette
Pimentos with Anchovies

Quiche Lorraine (no crust)
Escargots Bourgogne (Snails in Garlic Butter)

Soups
Consommé
Soupe à l'Oignon (Onion Soup)—no bread
Bouillabaisse (Fish Stew)

MAIN DISHES

Fillet of Sole Amandine (with Almonds)
Beef Stroganoff (Beef with Sour Cream)
Coquille Saint-Jacques
Veal or Chicken Cordon-Bleu (Rolled with Ham)
Coq au Vin (Chicken Stew with Vegetables and Wine)
Mousse à la Jambon (Ham Mousse)
Chateaubriand Bordelaise
Tournedos Béarnaises (Fillet of Beef)
Fromage Burger (Cheeseburger)
Chicken Soufflé

Salad
Mixed Green Salad

Vegetables
Champignons Grillés (Broiled Mushrooms)
Ratatouille (Vegetable Stew with Zucchini and
    Eggplant)
Épinard à la Crème (Creamed Spinach)
Salade Niçoise (String Bean Salad)

Desserts
Roquefort, Camembert, Gruyère, or Brie
Melon
Strawberries and Cream

Beverages
Demitasse
Coffee or Tea

Suggested Dinners from Greek Menu

Garides Ladolemono (Shrimp Cocktail with Lemon
  Sauce)
Moussaka (Lamb and Eggplant)
Melitzanosalata (Greek Salad)
Cheese Tray
Coffee

Soupa Me Lahano (Cabbage Soup)
Garides Tourkolimano (Shrimp Sautéed in Wine)
Salata Horta Vrasmena (Cooked Greens Salad)
Melon or Strawberries
Coffee

Greek Menu

Appetizers
  Garides Ladolemono (Shrimp Cocktail with Lemon
    Sauce)
  Donna Kebab (Meat Broiled on Spit)

Soups
  Soupa Me Lahano (Cabbage Soup)
  Kremithosoupa (Onion Soup—no bread)

Eggs
  Omeleta Me Sikotakia Poulion (Chicken Liver
    Omelet)
  Omeleta Me Loukanika (Sausage Omelet)
  Soufle Psari (Fish Soufflé)

Salads
  Salata Horta Vrasmena (Cooked Greens Salad)
  Melitzanosalat (Greek Salad)

MAIN DISHES

  Arni Sto Fourno (Roast Lamb)
  Arni Me Bamies (Lamb with Okra)

Kotopoulo Riganato (Chicken Oregano in Casserole)
Garides Tourkolimano (Shrimp Sautéed in Wine
    and Baked in Casserole with Feta Cheese, To-
    matoes, and Garlic)
Astakos Missiotikos (Broiled Lobster Tails)
Pasha Dava (Eggplant filled with Lamb and Cheese)
Glosses (Fillet of Sole)
Keftedakia Skaras (Mideastern-Style Chopped Beef
    and Lamb)
Shish Kebab
Moussaka (Lamb and Eggplant)—omit Béchamel
sauce

Desserts
  Strawberries
  Melon
  Cheese Tray

Beverages
  Coffee
  Tea

Suggested Dinners from Italian Menu

Pimentos and Anchovies
Veal Scaloppine al Marsala
Caesar Salad
Deep-fried Cauliflower
Cheese Platter
Espresso

Hot Antipasto
Chicken Francese
String Beans Marinara
Prosciutto and Melon
Cappuccino

Italian Menu

Appetizers
Clam Cocktail (ask for hot garlic)
Shrimp Cocktail (butter sauce instead of cocktail sauce)
Antipasto (hot or cold)
Pimentos and Anchovies
Provolone and Salami
Shrimp Scampi

Soups
Stracciatella
Consommé

Salads
Tossed Salad (oil and vinegar)
Caesar Salad (omit croutons)

MAIN DISHES

Seafood
Shrimp Marinara
Shrimp Fra Diavolo
Stuffed Shrimp (with Crabmeat)
Shrimp Salad
Scungilli Salad
Baked, Broiled, or Fried Flounder
Flounder Marinara
Lobster Tail Scampi
Lobster Fra Diavolo
Lobster Marinara
Tripe

Poultry
Boneless Chicken with Marsala Wine
Boneless Chicken with Butter Lemon Sauce
Chicken Francese
Chicken Scaloppine
Chicken Marinara

Veal
Veal Scaloppine al Marsala
Veal Scaloppine, Peppers, and Mushrooms
Veal Piccata with Lemon Butter Sauce
Veal Francese
Veal Marinara
Saltimbocca

Steak and Chops
Chopped Steak Marinara
Steak Pizzaiola
Steak Piccata

Pork
Sausages and Peppers
Fried Pork Chops

Vegetables
String Beans Marinara
Broccoli Sautéed with Oil and Garlic
Deep-Fried Cauliflower
Sautéed Escarole

Desserts
Strawberries with Wine
Prosciutto and Melon
Cheese Platter

Beverages
Espresso
Cappuccino (without sugar)
Coffee
Diet Soda
Dry White or Red Wine

Suggested Dinners from Spanish Menu

Gambas al Ajillo (Garlic Shrimp)
Gazpacho Andaluz (Cold Salad-Vegetable Soup)

Pollo a la Navarra (Chicken with Olives and
  Anchovies)
Spanish Melon
Expreso

Caracoles en Taza a la Borgoña (Snails)
Paella Valenciana
Ensalada Mixta
Fresónes con Salsa al Jerez (Strawberries with Sherry
  Sauce)
Coffee

Spanish Menu

Appetizers
  Mejillónes Salsa Verde (Mussels in Green Sauce)
  Caracoles en Taza a la Borgoña (Snails in Garlic
    Butter Sauce)
  Gambas al Ajillo (Garlic Shrimp)
  Melón con Jamón (Ham with Spanish Melon)

Soups
  Gazpacho Andaluz (Cold Salad-Vegetable Soup)
  Sopa de Pescado Almeria (Fresh Fish Soup)

Salads
  Ensalada Mixta (Tossed Salad)
  Olives and Anchovies

MAIN DISHES

Fish and Shellfish
  Carabineros Gaditanos (Spanish Prawns flavored with
    Brandy)
  Lenguado a la Asturias (Fillet of Sole Sautéd with
    Spinach and Mushrooms)
  Lubina a Horno Iberia Salsa Holandésa (Fillet of
    Striped Bass Hollandaise Sauce)
  Paella Valenciana (without rice) (Mixture of
    Chicken, Sausage, Seafood, and Vegetables)

Paella con Langosta (without rice) (same as above with lobster added)

Poultry and Meat
Pollo a la Navarra (Chicken and Tomatoes Sautéed)
Festónes de Ternera Don Quijote (Veal Scaloppine with Ham and Cheese)
Entrecotte Minuto (Minute Steak)
Entrecotte Parrilla (Prime Sirloin Steak)
Carre de Cordero Lechal (Rack of Baby Lamb)
Solomillo Parrilla (Salsa Béarnaise) Filet Mignon (Sauce Béarnaise)

Vegetables
Espárragos (Asparagus)
Judías Tiernas Salteadas con Almendras (String Beans with Almonds)
Espinacas Salteadas con Piñónes (Spinach Sautéed with Pine Nuts)

Desserts
Fresónes con Salsa al Jerez (Strawberries with Sherry Sauce)
Spanish Melon

Beverages
Expreso
Coffee
Tea
Dry Spanish Wine (not Sangria)

Suggested Dinners from Steak House Menu

Clams on Half Shell
Filet Mignon, Sauce Béarnaise
Spinach and Mushroom Salad
Cheese and Nuts
Coffee

Crabmeat Cocktail—Lemon Cream Dressing
Onion Soup
Rack of Lamb
Mixed Green Salad with Roquefort Dressing
Broiled Mushrooms
Strawberries and Cream
Coffee or Espresso

Steak House Menu

Appetizers
Prosciutto with Melon
Chopped Chicken Livers
Crabmeat Cocktail—Lemon Cream Dressing
Herring in Cream Sauce
Clams on Half Shell
Nova Scotia Salmon
Escargots à la Bourguignonne
Barbecued Chicken Wings or Legs
Melon
Meatballs

Soups
Onion Soup
Consommé
Lobster Bisque
Beef Broth with Meatballs

MAIN DISHES

Roast Prime Ribs of Beef
Sirloin Steak
Filet Mignon, Sauce Béarnaise
Broiled Lamb Chops
Broiled Pork Chops or Veal Chops
Porterhouse Steak
T-Bone Steak
Chateaubriand

Minute Steak
Tournedos
Fondue Bourguignonne
Brisket of Beef
Broiled Chopped Steak
Chicken or Veal Cordon-Bleu
Rack of Lamb
Broiled or Baked Chicken or Turkey
Broiled or Baked Fish, not stuffed
(Add 2 tablespoons mushrooms or onions on the
  side)

Salads
Garden Salad
Caesar Salad (eliminate croutons)
Spinach and Mushroom Salad
Mixed Green Salad

Vegetables
Broccoli with Cheese Sauce
Asparagus Hollandaise
Creamed Spinach
Broiled Mushrooms

Desserts
Cheese
Melon
Strawberries and Cream
Nuts

Beverages
Coffee or Espresso

Suggested Dinners from Dairy or Vegetarian Restaurant Menu

Vegetables and Sour Cream
Baked Flounder

Spring Salad
Cheese Tray
Coffee
Smoked Whitefish Salad
Spinach and Egg au Gratin
Blueberries and Sour Cream
Tea

Dairy or Vegetarian Menu

Salads
Vegetable Liver Salad
Salmon Salad
Sliced Egg Salad
Chopped Egg Salad
Chopped Herring Salad
Tunafish Salad
Sardine Salad
Smoked Whitefish Salad
Spring Salad

Eggs and Omelets
Two Eggs, Boiled, Scrambled, Fried or Poached
Shirred Eggs
Poached Eggs on Spinach
Omelet, Cheese, Mushroom, Onion, Fish
Chopped Spinach and Eggs

Cream Dishes
Pot Cheese and Sour Cream
Vegetables and Sour Cream
Fresh Strawberries or Blueberries and Sour Cream

Main Dishes (Fish)
Broiled Florida Pompano
Broiled Sea Bass
Baked or Broiled Red Snapper
Baked or Broiled Brook Trout

Baked or Broiled Salmon
Baked or Broiled Halibut
Baked, Broiled, or Sautéed Whitefish
Baked, Broiled, or Sautéed Flounder
Baked, Broiled, or Sautéed Sole
Pickled Herring

NOVELTY-TYPE DISHES

Spinach and Egg au Gratin
Vegetable Cutlet
Fried Eggplant Steak
Protose (Vegetarian Meat)

Desserts
Melon in Season with Prosciutto
Strawberries or Blueberries and Cream
Half a Grapefruit
Cheese Tray

Beverages
Coffee, Tea, or Diet Soda

We used certain products in this book because we found the carbohydrate count to be the lowest.

BAKEN-ETS: Distributed by Frito Lay, 1261 Zerega Ave., Bronx, N.Y.

D-ZERTA: Distributed by General Foods Corp., 250 North St., White Plains, N.Y.

EGG BEATERS: Distributed by Standard Brands, Inc., New York, N.Y. 10022

HUNT'S: Tomato products are packed by Hunt Wesson, Fullerton, California 92634

JANE'S KRAZY MIXED-UP SALT: Distributed by J. P. Simons Co., 1015 Chestnut Street, Philadelphia, Pa. 19107

LEA & PERRINS WORCESTERSHIRE SAUCE: Manufactured by Lea & Perrins, 1501 Pollitt Drive, Fairlawn, N.J. 07410

MAGGI'S SEASONING: Distributed by The Nestle Co., Inc., 100 Bloomingdale Road, White Plains, N.Y. 10605

NO-CAL SYRUP: Distributed by No-Cal Corp., 921 Flushing Ave., Brooklyn, N.Y. 11206

PAM: Distributed by Boyle-Midway, Inc., 685 Third Ave., New York, N.Y. 10017. Pam may be purchased in the cooking oil department of your supermarket.

WAGNER'S EXTRACTS: Distributed by John Wagner & Sons, Inc., Soyland, Pa. 18974

INDEX

ABOUT THE AUTHORS

DR. ROBERT C. ATKINS, author of the bestselling *Dr. Atkins' Diet Revolution: The High Calorie Way To Stay Thin Forever*, was born in Dayton, Ohio. He attended the University of Michigan and Cornell Medical College and was a resident at St. Lukes Hospital, in New York, before entering private practice as a cardiologist.

FRAN GARE and HELEN MONICA, two gourmet cooks, collaborated on the recipes for this book under the supervision of Dr. Atkins. A challenging task in and of itself, one has only to taste the recipes to see how well they met the task. Both Ms. Gare and Ms. Monica live in New Jersey.

How's Your Health?

Bantam publishes a line of informative books, written by top experts to help you toward a healthier and happier life.

Bantam Book Catalog

Here's your up-to-the-minute listing of over 1,400 titles by your favorite authors.

This illustrated, large format catalog gives a description of each title. For your convenience, it is divided into categories in fiction and non-fiction—gothics, science fiction, westerns, mysteries, cookbooks, mysticism and occult, biographies, history, family living, health, psychology, art.

So don't delay—take advantage of this special opportunity to increase your reading pleasure.

Just send us your name and address and 50¢ (to help defray postage and handling costs).

BANTAM BOOKS, INC.
Dept. FC, 414 East Golf Road, Des Plaines, Ill. 60016

Mr./Mrs./Miss_____
(please print)

Address_____

City_____ State_____ Zip_____

Do you know someone who enjoys books? Just give us their names and addresses and we'll send them a catalog too!

Mr./Mrs./Miss_____

Address_____

City_____ State_____ Zip_____

Mr./Mrs./Miss_____

Address_____

City_____ State_____ Zip_____

FC—9/76